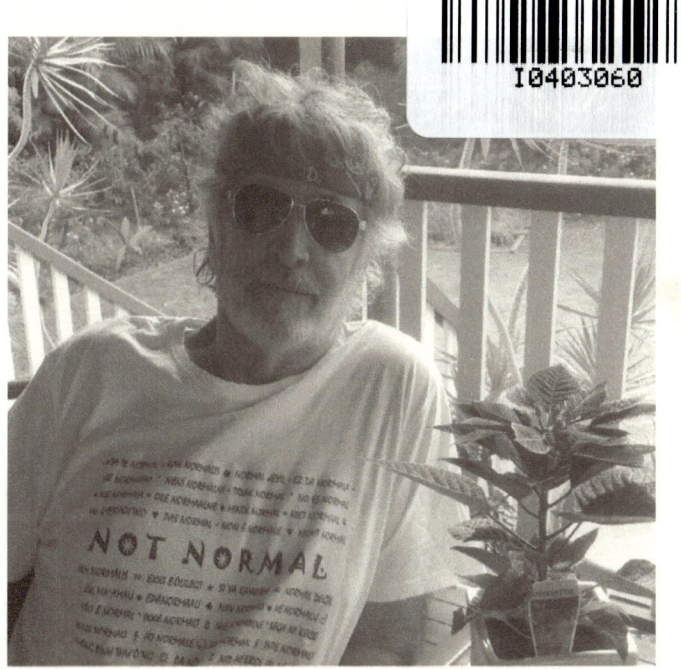

Jack Kregas was born in New England in the north east of the United States. After a stint in the US Army, he was discharged in Europe and the next forty years were spent skiing and living life to the max as well as creating several successful businesses.

After many winters in the Alps and summers windsurfing on Maui, Jack departed Switzerland for Maui full-time with his Australian wife and small daughter. Five years later, he moved to Australia with his family and became an Australian citizen.

Jack now lives in Brisbane and plays golf and tournament poker. After publishing his first book in 2015, the autobiography of his adventurous life, he has written another nine books.

OTHER BOOKS BY THE SAME AUTHOR

Fiction

Joey Moretti Thrillers

Mystical Glasses

Innocent Retribution

Contested Ransom

Decisive Sunset

Other Fiction

Choice Cruise Lines

Tall Tales – a Collection of Short Stories

Slick Justice

Non-fiction

It's All About Me and a few others

It's Not Only About Me

TALL TALES TWO

SHORT STORIES
TRUTH AND ADVICE

JACK KREGAS

Publishing Details

Tall Tales Two – Short Stories Truth and Advice by Jack Kregas

© Jack Kregas

The moral right of the author has been asserted. All rights reserved. Without limiting the rights under copyright restrictions above, no part of the production may be reproduced, stored in or introduced into a retrieval system, or transmitted in any form or by any means, (electronic, mechanical, photocopying, recording, or otherwise), without the prior written permission of both the copyright owner and the publisher of this book.

1st Edition 2018

Copyright: Jack Kregas 2018

This book is copyright

Apart from any fair dealing for the purpose of private study, research, criticism or review, as permitted under the Copyright Act, no part may be reproduced by any process without written permission.

This is a work of fiction. The events and characters in this book are fabricated from the imagination of the author. Some places and locations maybe real, others are not. Any similarity to any person living or dead is purely coincidental.

This book is dedicated to my friends who have had prostate problems, Glen T, John M, Bill M, Mike P, Charles M and Bill Van Atten who has shared his story in this book. The more men are informed, the greater the chance they have of an early diagnosis and a successful treatment. This was the motivation for this book.

Very special thanks to:

Dr. Alan Grigg, my General Health Practitioner practicing in Ipswich, Australia; and

Dr. Teng my Urological Surgeon practicing in the Ipswich region, Australia.

And as always, maximum gratitude to my editors, Susan and Megan, who have been with me from my first book and they inform me that after ten books their job has not gotten any easier. I agree writing is the easy part. Making it readable takes more talent than I have.

Contents

1. PEE-ved   (Truth)

2. Bill's Story   (Truth)

3. George   (Advice)

4. Not All Days Are The Same (Jack's truth)

5. Off The Grid   (Advice)

6. Being An Author   (Advice)

PEE-ved

Forward

In general, I do not like doctors. I don't trust them or the complete medical establishment. This is no particular reason for this. No bad experiences. I have been influenced by medical horror stories related by others, which made up my mind that doctors should be avoided. I have been fortunate enough to be healthy. All my experiences with doctors have been because of accidents, which for the most part, were my own doing.

At fourteen, a compound fracture of the right leg with bones sticking through my ski pants. Two weeks in a hip cast then an operation with two screws inserted to hold the bones together. Ten months later I was meant to go back to have the screws removed. They are still there today.

A torn meniscus in my left knee from skiing. No medical attention.

Broken ribs from falling on ski poles numerous times. No medical attention.

Two broken ribs in my back from coming off a mountain bike. X-rayed and went home.

Dislocated left shoulder in an avalanche. Doctor pulled it into place. Was skiing an hour later.

Dislocated right shoulder skiing. Same doctor, same result.

Ligaments torn and muscle torn away from left knee. X-rayed and told a reconstruction needed. Had therapy instead.

Informed that knees were bone on bone and needed replacement. No way Jose.

Informed that my PSA (Prostate Specific Antigen) was high. Was sent to a specialist who recommended a biopsy. The hell with that.

The following year a different doctor, same recommendation. This one was a female doctor who called me at my house and sent me letters telling me I had to sign-off that she had informed me I was in danger of prostate cancer and would not follow advice. I told her in her office that she had nice tits and I would like to invite her for dinner. I never heard from her again.

By chance, I went to Dr. Grigg for another matter. He was less than concerned and said to monitor it. I told him I preferred an erection and early death to a long life, limp. I have been going to him for check-ups for five years. He is my kind of doctor.

My PSA rose rapidly from one six-month period to the next. With a large prostate, as is common for men of a certain age, and a high PSA, Dr. Grigg recommended I see Dr. Teng, his choice of urologist. I made an appointment because I trusted his judgement.

From the start, I liked Dr. Teng. He explained the situation and possibilities. Have an MRI (Magnetic Resonance Imaging) to check the prostate. If it showed anything suspect, then have a biopsy. Depending on the findings, surgery may be required. Once you start with the MRI, you have to follow through. I told him I could live without knowing. He agreed to continue to monitor my condition every six months. My thinking was that if after eight years I had cancer, it was slow growing and I would die with it. Sex is more important to me.

I had no interest in having a biopsy and following through with surgery, if that was the call. I was not sick and had no intention of going into a hospital, a place that scared me and made me feel faint by the smell alone. I once visited a friend and could only manage to stay for less than five minutes. For me, it feels like a place of death and disease and is to be avoided at all costs. This is only my opinion and I appreciate the work the medical profession performs. It is just not a place for me.

August 2017, Brisbane

I'm restless again. I want to go on a trip. Every three months or so I feel like this. My latest book Tall Tales has been released and I can do a book signing in LA. I can visit my friend Charlie, watch the baseball playoffs, and visit a place I have never been. I decided that Zion Canyon and Bryce Canyon National Park were the places to go.

It is an easy drive from LA. I also planned to visit my friend Bill who was in Colorado. Bill has had an interesting life and has asked me to work with him on making his story into a book. This was to be a trip to could cover many objectives.

The next hurdle was to convince my traveling companion, Diane, to join me. She always has to check to make sure the timing doesn't clash with other commitments. Family, work, theatre, house, etc. I know in the end that she will give me some dates and I made plane reservations to fly to LA on 3 October.

We did some homework on Zion and Bryce canyons. Diane made hotel reservations and I decided to book a horseback ride in the red canyons near Zion. With Butch Cassidy's trail and hideout from when he first became an outlaw in this area, it appealed to me. A half-day ride was $99. A six-hour all-day ride with lunch was $120. Always a man looking for the best deal, I opted for the six-hour all-day adventure. The fact that neither Diane nor I had been on a horse in more than forty years didn't concern me. It sounded like fun.

The reason Diane and I have fun traveling is that she mostly goes along with my ideas. A few years ago she had her first attempt at snow skiing and then went back for a second year. What is the sense of going on a trip if it's not a new adventure and experience? Life is too short not to enjoy it while you can.

Tuesday, 3 October 2017

Gold class on Virgin gives us lounge access and other priorities, which makes flying much more comfortable. We boarded VA7, the direct twelve-hour flight to LA, bringing our own food. Airline food hardly qualifies as food. Just the smell of it makes me feel ill. The flight lands at seven o'clock in the morning local time. I try to sleep so I can arrive without jet lag.

I will not go on about how it can take up to two hours to clear customs. The system is worse than ever regardless of how automated they try to make it. Once out of the airport, it's onto a shuttle to pick up the rental car. I always book online with U-drive. They are half the price of all the others with all taxes included and the cars are sourced from the major players. It is then a thirty-minute drive to Malibu and my home away from home at Charlie's. Because of the time difference with Australia, we get to have Tuesday all over again, having more fun the second time around.

Wednesday, 4 to Thursday, 5 October 2017

There are traditions I have to follow when I arrive in the US. The first is to stock up on Häagen Dazs ice cream. I like Coffee, Strawberry and Vanilla Swiss Almond. None of the fancy flavors for me. Two of each will hold me for a day or two.

The next is a meal at Gilbert's Mexican restaurant on Pico. The waiters are the same as were there more than forty years ago, which was about the first time the place was recommended to me. The food has never changed. No-frills Mexican that, after finishing, you want to order the same meal again, to reassure yourself you weren't just dreaming how good it was. I have occasionally found Mexican food as good, but not better.

Taking in some shopping in Santa Monica, watching sport on television and talking politics with Charlie is a relaxing couple of days for me in LA.

For this trip, the plan is to drive to Mesquite, Nevada, a small town about 80 miles north of Las Vegas. It is 350 miles from LA, which takes about five hours, driving non-stop. We plan to stop at various shopping outlets along the way. Diane doesn't drive in the States. She did try it once near the Grand Canyon but prefers to be the navigator so we don't get lost. I don't mind driving, especially where you can still speed along without being busted by cops or cameras using road safety as an excuse for fundraising. It's a free feeling, rolling fast along roads through the desert.

Friday, 6 October 2017

We left LA around 7:00 am to avoid some of the traffic going to downtown LA. Driving in LA is a pure luck situation. There is always traffic. Sometimes it's fast, scary fast, across eight lanes or can be slow for no apparent reason. An accident will have you stuck in one place for hours. It takes an hour and a half to clear greater LA and be on the Interstate 15 to Vegas. I've done this drive many times and you can roll along at around 80 miles per hour if there aren't too many trucks.

The first stop is Barstow for coffee and then on to Primm located on the border of Nevada and California. A quick look in the outlet center and lunch at a Greek restaurant has us back on the road to Vegas.

When we came through, it was only five days since the mass shooting in Vegas. Fifty-eight people were killed and many hundreds injured. A memorial had been erected near the Mandalay Inn with the name of each victim displayed on individual white wooden crosses. Long lines had formed with people paying their respects to their friends and loved ones. Driving down the strip was surreal with most hotel billboards displaying the words - VEGAS STRONG.

An hour later, we arrived in Mesquite and checked into our hotel for the night.

Saturday, 7 October 2017

We were on the road again by ten o'clock the next morning, driving into Utah. The speed limit on the highway there is 80 miles per hour meaning around a hundred was the normal speed. Zion National Park was our first destination.

Parking in and near Zion is a problem especially on a weekend. We found a spot along the road several miles from the park. Fortunately, shuttlebuses cater for park visitors. From a nearby bus stop, we were taken by bus to the park entrance and the very long queue to get in. Using my charm and age, I scored a $20 pass for twelve months for all National Parks in the US. Cars and up to six passengers included. That saved us around $100 over the next few days.

Zion is impressive and well worth the visit. The National Parks Service provide another bus service, which travels along the river that cut the canyon millions of years ago. There are ten stops before it reaches the end of the canyon. You are able to get on and off, as you like. At each stop, there are hikes of various lengths and interests. We did a couple of these. Everywhere you looked were steep canyon walls of various shades of red depending how the sun hit them. Truly magnificent.

My advice to anyone visiting is to rent a bike, put it on the bus rack, go to the end of the canyon at stop ten and bicycle back. It's downhill almost all the way back, eliminating peddling and offering the possibility to stop and take photos whenever you want. Zion is 'a must see' if you're in the area.

We left Zion and drove about an hour to Cedar City where we spent the night. This is a small Utah town with an outstanding Mexican restaurant, Don Miguel. Sooo good and cheap.

Sunday, 8 October 2017

It was my birthday. To me, it is of little consequence as long ago I decided birthdays would no longer be counted. Your mentality, how you think and behave, is more important than any number. However, on this day I was seventy-five. Three decades of nonstop fun deserved to be noted, if not for any other reason than I never in my wildest dreams expected to live so long.

We drove to Bryce Canyon. This was a trip on a winding road through lava fields and forests, which at times had expansive views worth getting out of the car to appreciate.

Red Canyon is a few miles before the entrance to Bryce. This was our first view of the fantastic rock formations reaching up to the sky. We were excited, as our horseback ride into this canyon was booked for the next day. We did as most others, parked and took photos, as one formation was more stunning than the last.

I flashed my membership pass to the park officer and drove into Bryce Canyon. This canyon is between 8,000 and 9,000 feet (2,400 to 2,700 meters) above sea level. It has some of the purest air on earth with views that span 200 miles.

The Grand Canyon further south in Arizona, particularly the south rim, is breathtakingly spectacular from the first sighting. Bryce Canyon differs in the type of formations, the brilliant colors and the variety of intriguing landscapes seen from the viewpoints provided. It is famous for its unique geology, which consists of series of horseshoe-shaped amphitheaters carved from the eastern edge of the Paunsaugunt Plateau in southern Utah. Headward erosion, along with the dissolving power of rainwater have shaped the colorful limestone into bizarre shapes including slot canyons, windows, fins, and spires called 'hoodoos'. This type of erosion makes Bryce, despite its name, not technically a canyon.

We drove the 17 miles along the rim pausing often to take photos and enjoy the amazing geological structures and views of the Mars-like landscape. Words and photos cannot capture the natural beauty of this special place.

When we started, it was a warm eighty degrees, (27 Celsius). We were at almost 9,000 feet and by three in the afternoon, it started to cool. By the time we left the canyon and found our hotel/motel located outside the canyon park, it was cold.

We had booked in at the Bryce Canyon Pines Resort because they also had the horseback ride as one of the attractions. The motel was not cheap but another drawcard was that it had its own restaurant. Unfortunately, reservations could not be made and there was almost a two-hour wait to get a table. By now, it was very cold and we were hungry so we headed down the road and found an excellent café with good food and wine to celebrate my 'special' birthday.

Author's note: *Until now, this has read like a pleasant travel log through southern Utah. I would now like to warn those who may be squeamish that the following is a descriptive and factual account of how sometimes things don't go according to plan.*

Monday, 9 October 2017

The six-hour horseback ride was to begin at 9:00 am. We were up before seven, excited about the ride and surprised to see ice on the car windows. Outside the temperature was below zero with wind and clouds. We cleared the windscreen and drove 100 yards to the restaurant. Even with as many layers of clothing as we could wear, we were still freezing. The afternoon before a t-shirt was sufficient, now a t-shirt, a shirt, a sweater and a very warm Patagonia fleece was not enough. Diane had some more layers and had even cleverly brought gloves but was still cold.

The coffee had the taste of a tin bucket and I settled for that. Diane ordered eggs, which arrived after a prolonged wait. We paid and drove another 200 yards to the horse corral. Standing there in the freezing cold looking at the horses, I started to think that maybe the three-hour ride would have been a better choice. Another couple were there for the three-hour ride and after speaking with us decided to come with us on the day trip.

Our guide was a Marlboro Man look-alike. Steve, as he introduced himself, was a local rancher. With spats, boots, leather jacket, gloves and a neck scarf, he was the real deal. All that was missing was the six-gun. The horses were loaded into a float with us in the truck, to go to the entrance of Red Canyon, about 10 miles away. The very Red Canyon where Butch Cassidy hid out from many a posse.

The horses were unloaded and each of us were introduced to our mount. Mine was called Bean. Diane's called Sweetheart. They weren't at all interested in us. They looked tame enough to me but I was more concerned that I didn't have any gloves and my hands were freezing before we'd even mounted up. Steve said that within the first half hour we would adjust to the horse and be comfortable in the saddle. Of course, I believed him!

The sun was intermittent through the clouds, with some wind. It was cold, very cold. I rode holding the reins with one hand while the other was in my pocket, changing hands often. Steve led the way with the man and woman behind him followed by Diane, with me being the rear guard. Steve was right. We did adjust to the sway of the horse, and to some extent, it became more relaxed.

The horses were very sure-footed going up and down narrow paths. In some places the drop off was so far down, you thought it better not to look. By now, we figured that the horses were in control so it was best to just hang on to the reins and stay in the saddle while enjoying the ride and scenery.

It was two and a half hours before we took a break and dismounted. The temperature had warmed a little and the scenery was more than we could have imagined. We had climbed a mountain and according to Steve, we had two more to go over. Everyone used the makeshift toilet before mounting and again setting off.

Over the next couple of hours, we went up, down and around mountains before we stopped for lunch around 2:00 pm. There was the stone house without a roof said to be the actual hideout of Butch Cassidy. Steve shared its history and stories of Butch during lunch. I was surprised that I was not sore and had no trouble riding the horse. When I tried to pee behind a tree, it was next to impossible releasing only a few drops, even though I felt I had a full bladder.

After another hour in the saddle, I asked Steve if I could stop to take a leak. This time, try as I might, I was not successful. Back on the horse for another hour or so and we were back at the starting point at around four o'clock. I ran to a bush and tried pee. My bladder hurt. No success.

The drive in the truck back to the corral made it more painful.

We thanked Steve giving him a generous tip for his knowledge and professionalism. I drove like a maniac for the 300 yards to our room and into the toilet. No luck. I then told Diane of my discomfort. She checked Dr. Google to see what could be done.

I sat in a bath of hot water and wished to piss. No luck. I ran water over my fingers, same result. I paced the room, swearing and in pain. I pulled it, stroked it and begged it. It was not listening. At least four hours had passed since I had been able to relieve any pressure. I was now worried and in discomfort that was building by the minute. Every other minute, I would go to the bathroom and try to pee. For some reason this seemed to stop the hurt for a minute or two. Then the pain came again. It was no longer just discomfort. Dr. Google indicated that it was unlikely to improve.

At 6:30 pm, I asked Diane to call the hotel desk to find the whereabouts of the closest doctor or hospital. She was told there was a hospital in Panguitch, a small town 17 miles away. Diane called the clinic and the nurse advised that I needed to come in as soon as possible.

The car had ice on the windshield that had to be cleared. It was dark and there was a very cold wind blowing. I drove and fast. A speed sign said 65 miles per hour. I noticed I was going eighty.

"Shit, I just passed a cop on that side road. I bet he will be after our ass. Just what I need."

"Are you sure?" asked Diane hopefully.

Then I saw the flashing lights and heard the siren. My first thought was to outrun the cop but in a Hyundai Elantra, a bad idea. I pulled to the side of the road and stopped. The police car pulled in behind me about 30 yards away.

I opened the door and jumped out.

"Stay in the car," came a voice from the police vehicle.

I moved towards him with my hands in the air. I doubted he would shoot me with my hands above my head, although it did occur to me he might.

"I said stay in the car."

I walked towards the car.

The officer got out of his car, his hand on his hip, staying behind his open door.

"I'm on my way to the hospital. I'm in severe pain. I have some sort of blockage and can't piss. I know I was over the speed limit." I then turned and dashed off the side of the road, pulled out my penis and tried to pee.

The officer went to Diane's side of the car shinning a torch at her.

"He is in a lot of pain and has to get to the hospital," she told him.

As I came back to the car, "Can you escort us to the hospital?" I daringly asked as I danced up and down with a grimace on my face.

The officer said directly to me, "As of now you are detained. Let me see you driving license."

I got my license from the car and showed it to him.

"It's a Swiss license."

The officer who I thought to be about thirty-years old or less, glanced at it and handed it back. He stared at me.

"Okay. On your way but slow down. Drive in the limit to the clinic. Go ahead."

"Thank you. I will. Thank you again." I got back in the car quickly heading to the clinic.

"That was pure luck. I must have put on a good act or he could see the pain on my face. Maybe both. In any case, lucky."

With the address and the blue dot on the trusty Samsung tablet, Diane guided me to the clinic. I parked and galloped into the reception. While pacing and going back and forth to the toilet trying to urinate, Diane informed the nurse at reception of my situation. She remembered our call. I was told to lie down in a room on an adjustable operating bed. It was too painful to lie, so I sat. Every so often, I was up and off to the toilet hoping and now praying something would happen.

I was told there was no pill or quick fix. A catheter would have to be inserted. My mind raced. Having a tube stuck up my dick could not be pleasant. The only picture I could think of was from a book where in a Japanese prisoner-of-war camp they stuck a glass tube in the prisoner's dick and hit it with a hammer. I concentrated on the bladder pain instead. It was now close to 8:00 pm, almost eight hours without urinating properly.

"What the hell is the hold up?" I asked in a loud voice, probably more than once.

"I am a registered nurse. I will be looking after you. We will do a bladder scan to see how full it is."

"I am telling you how full it is. It feels like it is about to explode."

The registered nurse, a woman who I guessed to be in her late twenties, somehow didn't fill me with confidence. Another assistant wheeled in the bladder scanner. The registered nurse, who I shall call Jane, (not her name) tried to switch the machine on. She thought it might need a battery. They brought her a battery and she had no idea how or where to put it.

From little confidence, I was now extremely anxious that a person who didn't know how to work the machine, was about to stick a tube up my dick. If it had only been a haircut, I would have walked out. The amount of pain and danger I was in, did not afford me this option.

She finally got the machine to work and asked me to drop my pants. I lay back on the bed with my jeans around my ankles and my shoes on. She pulled down my jocks and spread transparent cream on my lower stomach to read my bladder.

"It's only about 700 mils. Your bladder can hold much more."

"Very comforting." I rolled my eyes at Diane who was standing beside me. Everyone else had left the room.

The clinic seemed to be empty; at least there were no patients that I could see. I pulled up my pants and went to the toilet, again trying to pee. *'Please let this happen now!'* I went back to the room.

"What the hell is going on? Where the hell are they, on a tea break? Please go out there and ask someone," I pleaded loudly.

"They are waiting for the doctor to come. It won't be long," Diane said, trying to reassure me about something she had no control over. Between the pain that was constant and the mental vision of a tube up my dick, I was in a state of panic.

At 8:36 pm, a young-looking doctor arrived. I don't recall his name. He had them take my blood pressure, which was by now, high and rising. The team surrounded me. The nurse opening packages and my pants again down around my ankles with my shoes still on was scaring me shitless as well as being in pain.

I lay back and tried to relax. Not possible. I felt the nurse take my penis.

"How painful is this going to be?" I asked.

"It will be uncomfortable. Don't worry I have done this hundreds of times. I never fail. I will put a catheter up your penis into your bladder and the pain will be relieved."

Her words were no comfort. Something told me I had not experienced anything yet.

I felt the catheter go into the head and screamed. My legs twitched as it went deeper.

"Fuck me, your killing me. Shiiit."

"Almost done," said the nurse as she pushed harder with the pain lifting me off the bed. But it wasn't close.

Sweat was pouring off my forehead. Diane asked for a wet towel and placed it over my forehead.

The nurse continued pushing the tube in. Nothing tender, just push and shove. I yelled out and swore, calling her unmentionable names. She was determined and kept on with my torture until with the doctor's advice she backed off. Before a second attempt, they decided to give me a shot of morphine but I didn't feel it had any effect at all. To an onlooker maybe it mellowed me out.

"I am sure you hate men and this is your revenge." There was no humor in my voice. I was angry and my first thoughts of her were haunting me. "She has no fucking idea."

Here I will let Diane give you her opinion of what she witnessed.

> *From when we arrived at the hospital, until treatment commenced, took quite a while and seemed even longer. The increasing pain, lack of action and reducing confidence exacerbated Jack's agitation.*
>
> *When they finally started, I was surprised at the minimal level of patient preparation, jeans at half-mast, shoes on and tube out ready to go.*
>
> *Presuming they knew what they were doing, I just held Jack's hands as I used to do for my children in medical situations,*

for comfort and to monitor their pain levels.

I was shocked that the procedure was shoving a tube up the penis while the patient was awake. We all heard the incredible pain Jack was feeling. Try as he might, he couldn't help lifting off the bed and raising the roof!

When I looked at what they were doing, I could see nothing but blood. How was this normal? The nurse kept going, jamming the tube in further with Jack yelling louder.

He was sweating profusely and I was worried he'd have a heart attack. I had seen his blood pressure levels on the chart before they started. They were already so much higher than his normal levels were. I asked for a wet towel but with no one concerned about this end of him, I found something myself.

Eventually the nurse realized she had not been successful in getting the tube into the bladder or the doctor had told her to stop. There was a lot of cleaning up to do and I got the distinct impression that the amount of bleeding was not normal. Jack now had more to worry about than just the pain from his bladder.

The nurse wasn't one to give in 'because she'd never failed' so was given permission to try again. This time they offered Jack some morphine, while insinuating he wasn't very tough. Despite knowing it wouldn't do much for the pain, Jack was willing to have anything.

Take two. This time before starting with the tube, she squeezed some gel into his penis. Whether it was a lubricant or anesthetic gel, I don't know. I do know that this step was not done the first time around. The second insertion was gentler but because of the prior damage was still very painful and Jack very vocal. The bleeding was slightly less but the outcome was the same.

The doctor, who had been cringing at the side of the room, advised that a scope was required for a successful insertion and Garfield Hospital did not have one.

The nurse appealed to the doctor, "I can do it. I've never failed. I will get it this time."

Reluctantly the doctor agreed for her to try again! Jack was not so keen. His profanities had increased following the morphine dose. The nurse repeatedly saying, "Hail Mary," did not help this. So

> *she had a third attempt, and as everyone except for the nurse expected, she failed.*
>
> *After all this trauma, Jack was in worse condition than when he arrived. After eight hours of not being able to urinate, damage can occur to the kidneys and a solution still had to be found. The only positive was that Jack must have a very sturdy heart.*

The third try was no more successful than the previous ones. My penis was now bandaged. Diane had told me I was bleeding so much she had to look away. I was wet with sweat and sat up on the bed. I pulled up my pants and stood up. It then hit me how much pain I was in from my full bladder, to say nothing of the burning inside my penis. I was extremely pissed off and paced around asking the doctor what the plan was now.

He said I would have to go the hospital in St. George that was 118 miles away. I gave him and the nurses a spray. He said we could drive there ourselves or they could have me taken in an ambulance. Diane and I discussed the options.

Driving ourselves meant that Diane would have to drive at night with me in a bad state and later have to deal with coming back for our gear at the hotel. So there was no real choice but for me to take the ambulance and for her to drive back to the hotel, pack, sleep, and join me in the morning. It meant she would have to drive. She realized this and gamely accepted the responsibility. I assured her that the drive would be no problem for her. For me things could not get much worse.

"Call the ambulance. You people sure fucked me up. I am far worse than I was before I came here. That nurse had no idea. Get me out of here." I paced and waited another twenty minutes for the ambulance.

It was 9:25 pm when I walked into the ambulance. It was less painful to sit than to lie down. There was a female driver with a guard in the front and a paramedic in the back with me. I was moaning and bitching.

"Turn on the siren and go faster I yelled to the driver."

"We're not allowed to do that. I can see you're in pain. I'll put this heat pad on your stomach, which may help. Also I can give you some more morphine."

"The last one didn't do much good but go for it. How long you been doing this?"

"My father retired after twenty-seven years last month. My mother has been in this job for sixteen and I have been doing it for eight and love it."

She injected the morphine into my arm. I checked my watch and felt every mile with my bursting bladder. "Are we there yet?"

"I don't want to be waiting around when we arrive. Can you arrange so they know we're coming and that they're ready for me?" I asked.

"I will call just before we get there. I'm like a bulldog. I piss them off sometimes but I will insure you get immediate attention. Hold on."

I thought, "*At last someone who knows what they are doing.*"

At 9:50, I received a text from Diane saying she was safely back at the hotel. She only saw three cars and a rabbit. She could drive in the US.

Just after 11:30 pm, we arrived at the Dixie Regional hospital in St George.

"I get in trouble if I don't wheel you in but I know you are better walking. Follow me in."

I followed her and thanked the driver who gave me a hug and wished me well. They were wonderful and I'm extremely grateful for the service they gave me.

I went directly to a room where two male nurses were waiting. It was now eleven hours since I had passed any water. The male nurses were friendly and joking.

"We will have you pissing in a minute. I never fail. First, we'll give you a shot to relax you and then I will inject plenty of lube with a numbing agent into your penis. Take of your pants and shoes and put on this gown."

"The last nurse told me she never failed and she had no idea. Why should I believe you? She didn't use any gel or numbing agent. I can't describe the pain. I'm not happy." I put on the gown.

"Don't worry I can do this. I have a bent catheter, which is far better for this process. She probably didn't have one like this. This shot will help and it will be uncomfortable. Are you okay?"

I watched the nurse. He had a laid-back attitude and was confident. I had no choice so took his word for it, thinking it cannot be worse than I had already experienced.

"You will feel the gel. Okay. That's done. I will wait a minute for the numbing agent to take hold and then your pain will be over."

"Why the hell didn't that bitch use gel and numbing agent? She just shoved it in."

There was no answer. The nurse was ready with the catheter. I could feel it going in. Not pleasant but nothing like before. He took it slow and gentle. I thought that only a man could imagine how that tube will feel like going up his dick. I didn't scream but squirmed.

"I am sorry. That woman really butchered you. I can't get it into your bladder as she's made a false passage. Instead of going into your bladder, she punched a hole in your urethra on the path of least resistance for the catheter. I'll have to call the urologist. He'll make a decision. I can say he will no doubt have to take you upstairs and use a scope."

"Hey man, you did your best. I appreciate how you went about it. When will the urologist get here?"

"We'll call him at home. It won't be long."

I was left alone on the bed. Make pain your friend filled my head as I tried to figure out what went wrong. *"Sure, I have a large prostate, which is normal for my age. At times, I've not had the strongest stream and in the last year it became somewhat less. I never thought about it for more than a minute. Now it's clear that six hours on the horse traumatized my prostate. The swelling strangled the urethra thus blocking the flow. It should have been something that I was made aware of or warned about but the focus has always been on prostate cancer. Maybe I should have known this before booking the ride. That's not my style and never has been. Go for the fun and worry about it later. Age may be a factor in reassessing that line of thinking. Now where is that doctor?"*

1:35 am Tuesday, 10 October 2017

The urologist arrived and introduced himself. He carried a silver box with him. I glanced at the box as he opened it. It held silver instruments that, to me, appeared to be from the middle ages. I was by this time in far too much pain to be worried about a bit more. The two male nurses were by his side.

"I had no luck at all," advised the nurse who had tried.

"Someone made a mess of you. A real butcher job," the urologist exclaimed as he tried with a catheter. "She created a false passage and now that's where the catheter goes each time. I'll have to use a scope to get the catheter into your bladder. Take him upstairs to the OR."

The doctor turned to me and said, "We will take you upstairs and put you out in order to use the scope to find the entrance to your bladder. Not long now and you will feel a lot better."

"Whatever you say," was my only reply.

I took my phone and sent a message Diane. It was 2:15 am. The morphine had affected some of my fine motor skills and I didn't have any glass with me! The text translated said, 'going to operate because girl fucked up in Garfield.'

They came with a bed on wheels, put me onto it and brought me upstairs. A mask was put over my mouth and nose. The lights went out.

I blinked and opened my eyes. "I guess I'm not dead," I said.

"No. Would you like some ice? Your mouth may be dry."

I turned to my right to see a stunning woman in black. "You look great. How old are you?"

I saw her smile. "I'm forty-one."

"You look twenty to me. Thanks for the ice."

I had a bag strapped to my leg. I felt no pain and did not feel any effects from the anesthetic. It was not long before I was moved into a private room. I asked for my phone and messaged Diane at 3:27 am, 'had operation in theatre' or words to that effect.

I then phoned her to say it all went well, no pain now and I would see her in the morning. I told her to have a safe drive. I thought the drive might be stressing her out so it was probably not very sensible to call when she would be sleeping. Blame the drugs!

I then went to sleep until just before 7:00 am. I sent a text to Diane to ask if she had left yet. I felt good and was ready to get out of there. My text had woken Diane. She had not slept much but let me know she was now up but would be a bit later than expected.

Diane's thoughts about the drive.

When you have to do something, you just deal with it. I actually operate very effectively in these circumstances, having had lots of practice. I go into a super practical, methodical mode. And that's what I did.

I made myself very aware of having to be on the right-hand side of the road because leaving the hospital at 9:30 pm meant there were few cars to give me guidance. It did however allow me to get used to the different driving at a sensible speed.

Back at the hotel, I packed up everything and had a cup of tea, courtesy of Garfield Hospital. The receptionist there was the loveliest person so far in this whole ordeal and allowed me to use a special tearoom, as I hadn't had any food or drink since we were at Butch Cassidy's house.

I checked the maps on the tablet and planned the 135-mile route to St. George and the hospital. Knowing which lanes to be in and the exits to take, made me feel I could tackle the speeds on the highways.

I showered and was having trouble falling asleep when Jack called at about 3:30 am. He had previously sent a couple of messages, which needed some decoding!

Talking to him and knowing that they had sorted him out, made it easier to relax. I fell asleep thinking that it was only one day after turning seventy-five and problems had already started!

I planned to get up at 6:00 am, pack the car and have some breakfast at the restaurant before heading off. I was in a deep sleep when Jack sent a message just before seven o'clock. I jumped into action and let him know I would be on my way soon. I was annoyed because I had wanted to have some breakfast and get on the road early while it was quiet.

The first problem was that the car was covered in ice; even the water bottle inside the car was frozen. I packed the car, drank some tea, and scraped off the ice. The next problem was the restaurant, as usual, was full and there was a queue for breakfast. There was no way I was going to wait. Our leftover provisions from the ride, an apple and some crackers would have to keep me going. I handed in the key just before eight o'clock, got no reaction from reception when I told them some of the story, sent a message to Jack and hit the road.

It was a great drive. Once I reached the Interstate 15, speed limit 80 mph, I had adapted to the car and the right-hand lanes. I cruised behind a small truck at eighty for half the trip. It just felt like driving at sixty in Australia. St. George was busy but I followed the signs and found the hospital car park.

It was good to see Jack in a much-improved state, happy and eager to go. Then came the bombshell that I would have to keep on driving. I hadn't thought past getting to St. George but it was clear that Jack was not allowed to drive. Anyway, we just got on with it, driving through Vegas and onto Primm, where we stayed the night.

It found it more harrowing driving in and around the cities with so many cars going in all directions, still at high speed. I won't talk about trucks. So I can drive in the States. I just need a good navigator!

The hospital and staff at St. George were outstanding. Besides being very attentive, they explained the use of the bag and tubes down my leg. With my jeans on and telephone in hand, there were no bad effects from the previous night that I could detect, except for the bag strapped to my leg and the torment dealt me in Garfield fresh on my mind.

The urologist came by and told me the nurse had made a false passage by using too much pressure in trying to insert the catheter. The damage would heal in time. I discussed that we would be in the States another week before returning to Australia.

He informed me the catheter normally would be taken out after a couple of days. Since I had additional damage, it would be okay for me to wait until I got home and have my doctor do it. The extra days with the catheter would give it more chance to heal and hopefully allow my bladder to work as it should. There would be some bleeding for a few days. He gave me antibiotics to take over the next week to prevent any infection. He shook my hand and wished me well.

Diane messaged at 7:53 to tell me she was leaving the hotel and arrived safely at St. George hospital at 10:30 am.

While I was waiting, I thought about what we could do for the next week. The plan had been to drive to Colorado and visit my friend Bill to work on his book. He had sent me pages of information and I wanted to go through it with him, discussing the details and timelines of when things happened.

The drive, which would be at least seven hours and then a long drive back to LA, no longer held my interest. A few days in Vegas could be fun. I would wait and see what Diane thought.

PEE-ved

When Diane arrived, I was ready to leave the hospital. A man had arrived from the pharmacy and given me the tablets the doctor had prescribed. I paid him $59 with a credit card. I thanked the nurses and left the hospital, walking with a strange gait because of the bag strapped to my leg.

"Any problems driving? You did great. I told you driving here was no big deal."

"I had to get used to the speed. On these Utah roads, it was no problem," she informed me.

"I will sit back and let you drive. Let's head towards Vegas and decide what to do. I told Bill it was too far and that we would not be able to visit him. We will arrange something at another time. I think the best idea is to go back to Charlie's and stay there until we leave for Australia. I feel okay but with this bag and the possibility of an infection, maybe that is the best idea."

"Sounds okay to me, except for me driving. California's roads are not so good and Vegas is crazy."

"Did you pay anything in Garfield? I didn't pay here. I guess they will send the bill. The way they treated me, maybe I'll sue?"

"I don't think they took a credit card number in Garfield. The woman there who was very nice told me that maybe they wouldn't charge. We will have to wait. When I think of what I saw that nurse do, it sickens me."

"I have no pain now and feel no effects from the anesthesia. I don't feel like stopping in Vegas. Let's go to Primm and spend the night there. Then talk to Charlie and go on to LA."

Wednesday, 11 October 2017

We stayed overnight in Primm. Diane drove through Vegas without any problem but said she would not drive into LA. She would drive to Barstow and we would change. The bag tied to my leg was hard to get used to, mostly because the tube coming out of my penis was uncomfortable. Every time I peed, it burned. There was blood in the urine and leakage. I had to live with this for the next week until we returned to Brisbane. It made me feel incapacitated. I had to go into a toilet cabin to disconnect the bag and empty it.

I had asked the urologist at the hospital what would happen once the catheter was removed. He said that most likely I would be able to pass water. By then, the prostate would have had time to recover from the trauma of the ride. One of the tablets he gave me was an anti-inflammatory and another was to shrink the prostate but it takes months.

His last words were, "It will be okay."

I had to believe him, as I could not cope with the thought of another tube up my dick.

I called Charlie and let him know we would be back early, as we wouldn't be going to Colorado. He was happy to have someone to talk baseball to during the play offs. His home was like my second home. I had been staying there for forty years. If it was not for this, I doubt if I would ever go to LA. The house on the cliff in Malibu was the perfect base. It now would be a place to chill before returning to Australia.

Charlie and I have a long history of good times and adventures in Verbier, Aspen and other places. Not only is he a true friend but I owe him big time for letting me stay at his house. Thanks Charlie!

Thursday, 12 to Wednesday, 18 October 2017

"How come you guys are back so early?" Charlie asked.

I dropped my pants showing him the tube going down my leg into the bag. Charlie was surprised then laughed as I recounted the story.

"Shit happens. I don't blame the horse. I blame it on getting old."

The next five days were spent watching the baseball, US politics, eating Mexican food and plenty of Häagen Dazs ice cream.

I had a book signing at the Pipe and Thimble bookstore with fellow author Mark Fine, promoting my new book, Tall Tales, my first attempt at short stories. I made no mention of my ordeal.

We left at 11:50 pm on 18 October on the thirteen-hour Virgin flight to Brisbane, losing a day and arriving at 7:00 am on 20 October. I slept most of the way not bothering to get up and empty the bag. When we landed, not only was the bag full but there was a lot of blood in it.

Friday, 20 October 2017

The bleeding had almost stopped during the past week. Now seeing so much blood, I was frightened. I called my doctor, Dr. Grigg and made an appointment for the afternoon. Diane thought I should have got up and emptied the bag during the flight. I couldn't see how this made any difference and didn't agree. Dr. Grigg referred me to go to my urologist, Dr. Teng, to obtain the best advice. Both doctors have offices in the same area, so I went from one office to the other.

"Sorry, but Dr. Teng is not available today. You can see another urologist, Dr. Ali."

"Okay. I think I should see someone."

I waited and eventually Dr. Ali invited me into his office. Dr. Ali was a friendly guy who at seventeen went to New York and sold t-shirts on the streets. He was very proud of this. The ability to sell was still with him. He made me an appointment at a private hospital in a week's time, to take out the catheter and told me about a procedure called greenlight laser surgery.

GreenLight Laser Prostatectomy (or Photo-Selective Vaporization of the Prostate – PVP) is a relatively new procedure for the treatment of urinary blockages caused by the non-cancerous enlargement of the prostate (otherwise known as Benign Prostatic Hyperplasia or BPH).

He gave me a brochure about this procedure where a laser is used to trim the prostate allowing the urethra to have more room for urinal flow. I left somewhat confused and feeling I had been sold a deal more than having a specialist appointment.

According to Dr. Ali, the blood in the urine from the flight was normal. Too much sitting, the air pressure or that the tube had been in for more than a week could also have caused it. Over the next few days, it cleared up.

Saturday, 24 to Sunday, 25 October 2017

Prior to the trip, I had paid for a table at a two-day book fair in Brisbane. I sold some books and enjoyed meeting other authors during the weekend. A tube and bag of piss strapped to your leg should not stand in the way of selling books.

Monday, 23 October 2017

Since Friday, I had not been feeling confident about the whole Dr. Ali arrangement so I called Dr. Teng and he slotted an appointment in for me for the next day.

Tuesday, 24 October 2017

Dr. Teng heard the story from the beginning. He told me what I already knew, that I had a large prostate. The horseback ride aggravated it, as would a long bike ride. Blood in the urine after what I had been through was normal. He outlined a plan. On Thursday 26 October, Diane or I could take the catheter out at home, an easy undertaking, which is virtually painless. After this, I should be able to pee. Because Dr. Teng was going to be out of the state, he advised me what to do if it didn't work. I live near a large hospital so he wrote a letter for me to take to the Emergency Department if required.

Wednesday, 25 October 2017

I called and cancelled the appointment with Dr. Ali. After speaking with Dr. Teng, I was far more confident. Taking the catheter out at home was already saving me $1,000. It always pays to have a second opinion. I was apprehensive and excited about taking the catheter out. It had been in for over two weeks. My penis was swollen, sore, and unhappy. Diane was confident it would all be over in the morning.

Thursday, 26 October 2017

The catheter came out painlessly at 7:00 am. What a relief. I stood in the shower, enjoying the hot water flow over me with no tube or bag. I then began to drink water. A liter an hour. Around ten o'clock, I actually passed a stream of urine, weak and burning but it made me happy. A relief came over me. Maybe, just maybe, the trials of the last eighteen days were over.

After two hours, the light stream was now only drops. I drank more water and hoped. By late afternoon, there were still drops. My confidence was starting to wane. It should be getting better but instead, was getting worse. I cooked dinner and by 6:00 pm, I was in some discomfort. It was the night of 9 October all over again except now I knew what was in store for me, more pain. I was in trouble.

I told Diane I would have to go to the hospital. We went to the emergency room and waited. My bladder was painful. I knew the feeling well. After filling out the paperwork, I was shuffled from one nurse to another until finally I was examined. A nurse was going to insert another catheter but I demanded they get a urologist. I was told the urologist would have to be called in from home. History repeating itself, this time in Brisbane and not Utah.

I knew it would not be as bad as Utah but as I knew what was coming I was became progressively more uneasy, panicked, as I waited with increasing pain. My thoughts were, *"shit I have lived too long. Live too long and suffer."* I did realize, compared to some in the hospital, I was being a candy-ass. Thinking of blood flying from my already sore and inflamed dick filled my mind and I was feeling sorry for myself.

Dr. Tam, a female urologist arrived and told me what I didn't want to hear. She would put in another catheter. She said she had done hundreds and it would be no problem. Those were the worst words I could hear and made me want to swear and call her a fuckwit. I didn't like her abrupt bedside manner and now she had spoken the same words as the others. I was living proof that my experience meant nothing. I tensed for pain.

Having the letter from Dr. Teng was very useful, as Dr. Tam had trained and worked with him. She was informed of my history, the false passage and the difficulties others had had in inserting a catheter. Her manner softened. Understanding the obstacle that faced her, she took appropriate action to insure she didn't fail and to minimize my discomfort.

First, she gave me morphine and then Fentanyl, an opiate fifty to a hundred times more powerful than morphine. Following this, a generous quantity of lubricant was squeezed into the head. She then used a wire to guide the catheter. In spite of her professionalism, Fentanyl or not, it still hurt. Maybe the drugs eased the pain but when you are aware of the possible severity of the pain in your mind that is what you feel. Fuck, shit, and all their word friends followed as the catheter went in. I give her full credit. She was the only one, not using a scope, to insert the catheter in the proper place and on her first attempt.

While discussing the next steps, I asked her opinion of the greenlight laser surgery. She advised that the Royal Brisbane Hospital didn't have the funds for the equipment to do this. They only did the Transurethral Resection of the Prostate (TURP).

Her last words were, "Get this sorted before you take any more trips."

I thanked her and left the hospital with a tube and bag in place until 7 November. At that time, I would come back, have the catheter out and have my flow measured. If it was satisfactory, I was clear. If not I would have to make a date for surgery.

Friday, 27 October to Tuesday, 7 November

The next day, I had trouble getting out of bed. I felt like I had a hangover and then some. More like I was drugged. I blamed it on the Fentanyl. I went back to bed and slept. When I smoked dope, I enjoyed the high, the munchies and the discoing all night long. How this made me feel left me wondering why anyone would take these opiates. In 2016, there were over 59,000 overdose deaths in the US. Over 1,800 in Australia. Scary figures and more frightening totals.

This time there were some improvements in the set up with the bag attached to my thigh instead of my ankle. Because the tube was shorter and thinner, there was less movement and less irritation to my penis. The tube hooked to a night bag so I didn't have to get out of bed at night.

Now I had almost two weeks with a catheter and full-time worrying about what would happen if it didn't work on 7 November. The best thing to do was visit my friend, Dr. Teng. I listened and he gave me confidence. This doctor really cares about his patients.

I asked about the greenlight laser surgery, and he explained it. It was the best possibility for an enlarged prostate. If it didn't work, there was the TURP, a procedure where an electric knife is used. This involves more bleeding and a longer hospital stay. Dr. Teng said that these were only options if, after the catheter was out, I couldn't pee. He would be able to do the laser surgery in November, if it was necessary.

He was optimistic that by the seventh, there would be sufficient improvement from the trauma and it would work again. For now, I should be positive that I would pee okay when the catheter came out. Using the theory of preparing for the worst, he made a tentative booking for greenlight laser surgery for the 15 November. I signed the paper work for the operation before leaving the office just in case.

At home, the more I thought about it, the more I was of the mind to forget about taking the catheter out on 7 November because if it didn't work, another one would have to be put in until the fifteenth. Why not just have the operation? It seemed to make more sense. Another out and in of a catheter was something I particularly wanted to avoid.

I sent a message to Dr. Teng to ask what he thought. He called me back that evening saying that in his opinion there was more than a seventy percent chance that I would be able to pee. His advice was to go ahead with the removal on the seventh. He knew I really didn't want the operation and maybe was trying to save me the worry. I told him I would let him know my decision.

In the meantime, Diane was asking Dr. Google all the pertinent questions and accumulating information on the laser surgery and TURP. She shared the information with me. We discussed the pros and cons. The more I knew, the more comfortable I would feel with whatever was to happen in the future. The laser procedure meant one night in the hospital after the operation, some bleeding, which could last up to five weeks, discomfort with burning while urinating, and no sex for at least a month. The other negative side effects that happened in a very small percentage of cases, I didn't worry about.

My mind was not made up as to what to do. Have the catheter out and see, or go straight to surgery. It changed by the hour. I kept thinking, based on the past month, I would not be able to pee and then need the surgery. I was beginning to accept that. At the same time, why not give it another try, and maybe, hopefully, not need the operation.

I confirmed I would be at the hospital on 7 November, hoping for the best. That way every possibility had come into play. I would go the distance. In the end, if I couldn't pee, how much more torture would another catheter be. I knew the answer to that!

Tuesday, 7 November 2017

The appointment was for 9:00 am. I didn't have to wait. A very friendly nurse took out the catheter. She said to drink a lot of water and wait around. They would measure the amount of urine passed and at the same time how much was left in my bladder. After three times, if more was passed than left in my bladder, I could leave and no surgery would be necessary. After ten o'clock, I peed 200ml and 200 remained in my bladder. It was not a strong stream.

I was on high as at least I was able to pass some. I went to the coffee shop in good spirits. An hour later another 200ml but about 250 was left behind. The nurse was not impressed. She said to keep trying but had told Diane it didn't look good. Half an hour later nothing! I was depressed, not so much that it didn't work or that I would now face surgery, but now I would have to have another catheter. Would this never end?

I had drunk liters of water that filled my bladder. The familiar pain of not being able to pee returned with a vengeance. Again, I paced around the office. The nurse was very nice and I discovered she had worked with Dr. Teng for many years.

"I will try to put the catheter in and if I have any problems I will have to get a urologist to use a scope to do it."

To me that translated as two tries. I lay back on the bed and thought what does not kill me makes me stronger. Prepare for the hurt. The lubricating gel and numbing agent hurt. There was no morphine or injections. She was gentle with the catheter and quick to realize that it was not going where it should but into the false passage. She withdrew the tube and said she would call for the urologist and arranged for a scope.

He would be here soon. I laughed. The same well-rehearsed lines that really meant I would wait in pain. It was after 1:00 pm when the urologist arrived. A good-looking Greek doctor with a $100 shirt and a dapper tie. He was all business with a strained bedside manner. I waited while the scope was brought into the room and set up.

The urologist was now ready for his try using the scope and he hit the mark. Diane could clearly see the false passage on the screen. There is no need to explain the pain but I will say it was less than I imagined it was going to be. I thanked the nurse and the doctor and left the hospital at 2:00 pm as the Melbourne Cup horse race started. This is the most famous horse race in the country. I listened on the radio as Diane drove me home. It started on horseback and ended listening to a horse race.

I felt somewhat relieved. The future was now clear. No more catheter insertions while conscious. The next procedure would occur while I would be asleep and feel nothing. I had prepared my mind for this outcome. Fix it once and for all and move on. I had to wait a week until 15 November.

Wednesday, 8 to Wednesday, 15 November

It was now a month since this saga began. I am most grateful to Diane to being there with me providing support. Without her, giving up would have been easy. It had been a month with a catheter and would continue for another week. The present one was by far the most comfortable. Why could I have not had one like this at the beginning? This story has been written to ask these questions and forearm readers with knowledge and information.

After nine insertion attempts by six different people, I now had my third catheter with only one being successfully inserted without a scope.

It all stemmed from the first non-professional, inexperienced, (my idea, regardless of what she said), and pigheaded nurse who went on trying when she should have stopped. Why didn't she use lubricant and numbing gel? Why was she so determined when she had clearly failed? Why did the doctor looking on not say 'enough is enough'?

Was I unlucky, or was my original lack of trust in most doctors and the medical system in general, justified? Probably some of both. In any case, for those reading this please, whatever you have, obtain more than one opinion. If you don't feel confident, find someone who you are happy with. It can really be life, lots of pain or even premature death.

I reported to Dr. Teng that the attempt had failed so I would see him on 15 November. I was satisfied that I was in good hands, which put me at ease. I only had two concerns about the procedure. One was that I wanted the laser to work and not have to have the TURP. The second was I did not want a spinal block. I had read that normal anesthetic drugs used could remain in your body for up to a year. I did not want this but saw no way to avoid it. I could only ask for less drugs.

The procedure would not take place if I didn't pay the doctor, the anesthetist, and the hospital in advance. This may sound strange to some and health systems vary in all parts of the world. In Australia, there is Medicare, which means medicine is free until it's not. Through Medicare, if you need a knee replacement, you can wait for months or years, and have no choice of the doctor. You get who they give you.

There is also the possibility of having private health care, which you pay for. Of course, there is an excess, which you pay anytime use claim the insurance. I am not a believer in insurance. After years of driving without car insurance and no home insurance, I never considered health insurance. Fortunately, I have not needed it. Medicare covers visits to my normal doctor and gives partial refunds of what I pay for my urologist. It is possible to use your choice of doctor in a public hospital in Queensland but you have to pay the majority of the doctor's fee while only paying a small amount for the hospital.

I paid for everything in advance and was less out of pocket than if I had private healthcare, leaving me way ahead. In any country, I believe if you are in trouble with the law or have health problems and do not have money, you go to jail or die. Sad but true.

The week went by without anxiety. I knew what was to happen. I had only to hope it went well.

Wednesday, 15 November 2017

I was to be at the hospital at 11:00 am. The procedure was scheduled for 2:00 pm. I waited an hour before being led into a room to wait again while filling out one form after another and surrendering my clothes for a robe and an attractive red cap. The robe was one of those where your ass hangs out like Jack Nicholson's in the movie, 'Something's Gotta Give'.

Eventually, I was taken into a room where they did an electro-cardiogram (ECG) to see if my heart had any problems that would not withstand the procedure. No problem, it had survived Garfield. Diane departed saying she would see me when it was over. I hoped so. Next, into another room, where a nurse asked the same questions again.

"This is the third time I have been asked the same questions, name, age, why am I here, etc. Why is that?"

"We don't want to make a mistake and mistakes do happen. Not today but when it's busy and crazy in here. We have to be sure we are doing the right operation on the right person."

"I appreciate that."

Dr. Teng came into the room looking very different in his blue operating-room attire.

"Do you have any questions?"

"I don't think so. You know I want the laser. If you can do that I am happy."

"I will do my best."

I believed him. That was what counted.

Next came a young doctor who was in charge of the anesthetics.

"I will be in charge of you. Do you have any questions?"

"Only no spinal."

"No spinal. Understood."

"Less drugs, no opiates."

He laughed. "We have to make sure you don't wake up until it's over."

He wheeled me into an area adjoining the operating room and gave me a shot. Goodnight.

The operation lasted two hours and fifty-seven minutes. I woke up sometime after that, went back to sleep and woke up in a ward after 6:00 pm. There was a catheter in, which I knew would come out in the morning. I felt good. No pains and preferred to go home but that was not going to happen until sometime the next day. My guess was that the laser surgery had worked. I awaited word from Dr. Teng. In the meantime, Diane went home. I refused any hospital food, which looked like airplane food but didn't smell as bad. I avoid both.

I slept with frequent wake-ups caused by bells ringing and the noise of movement in hallways. There were three others in my ward, all friendly. It was a recovery ward with people there for a day or so before being discharged. It was in a wing well away from the area of the hospital where there were sick people. I liked that as I thought my chances of infection were somewhat less.

The nurses were very attentive taking my temperature and blood pressure every couple of hours and keeping me awake. They regularly checked the bag that was attached to the catheter, emptying it when necessary. I slept the best in the morning.

Thursday, 16 November 2017

I woke at eight ready to leave. I knew that was not going to happen at once. They would come and take out the catheter and then monitor how much I peed for at least three hours or until I was peeing and leaving less in my bladder than I peed. I knew the pack drill. This time I was confident.

The registered nurse was about thirty. Her assistant was working part-time and part-time in university. She was young, from Sri Lanka and shy. She was instructed to take out the catheter and was embarrassed. I leapt at the opportunity.

"Are you sure you can do this without me screaming?" I asked.

She hesitated then smiled nervously.

"Have you done this before? Am I the first you are here to torture?"

Again she stopped. The registered nurse knew exactly what I was doing and told her assistant, "Don't let him bother you and just go on with it."

"I am just giving her training for when she encounters someone difficult."

Out came the catheter.

"Now you have to drink and when you can, pee into that bottle. We'll measure it and what remains in your bladder. It will take a couple of hours to see how you are going," the registered nurse advised.

Now it was all up to me. I had to be able to pee to get out of the hospital. I drank a glass of water.

"How you feeling?" asked Dr. Teng.

"As soon as I pass the pee test, I am ready to get out of here. I feel good. Some burning that's all. I guess you accomplished it with the laser?"

"Yes, I wanted this to work. I scheduled you at the end of the day so I would have plenty of time. I started slowly with very low power and gradually increased it as I went along. It took almost three hours but the result is as good as it could be."

"I really appreciate your skill and looking after me so well."

"With the laser procedure, you can usually tell in the first five minutes if it will work."

"You didn't tell me that before."

"I was intent on making this a success. This is my specialist field. When there is a challenge, I am on top of it."

"I am lucky to have you. Thank you again."

"I've given you antibiotics against any infection. That's what you have to be careful with now. Keep taking the antibiotics you have for another two weeks. If there are any problems, call me immediately. I want to see you in about six weeks so please make an appointment."

"Now I only have to pee."

"You will be better than ever. Don't worry."

I turned to Diane and said, "How lucky was I to have him. Someone else and I would have been in the too-hard basket and had TURP. I am very happy. Just goes to show it pays to choose the best doctor."

Diane agreed as I headed for the toilet with a bottle in hand. There was some success and plenty of burning although in the past I had felt worse. 150ml in the bottle and about the same amount left in my bladder. I drank and waited for the next try.

The next time was about the same. I ran my fingers under warm water to try to trick my bladder into responding. A rough description of the bladder is a sack controlled by muscles. In the last month with the catheter, it had stretched and, with no need to try to push, the muscles became lazy. Now I had to wake them up. Push you bastards! Force it down the tube!

The nurse gave me a tip. Wait ten minutes and then try again. We will count the two tries as one. It will show a better result. That was a great tip. I grabbed the bottle and was back in the toilet. More in the bottle and less in the bladder. Now that was to be excited about.

Two hours later, there was again more in the bottle and less in the bladder. I asked for my clothes and dressed. A doctor who worked with

Dr. Teng came by with two nurses and checked my results.

"You know you can't leave until we are sure that you are voiding your bladder. It makes no sense to send you home and have you back this evening. You have to wait until we are sure." He left the ward.

I tried again with a better result. I saw the doctor in the hall by the station and went up to him.

"It's going better. I'm fine. I can leave now."

The doctor was young and avoided my statement, instead asking me about skiing. How he knew I skied I had no idea. Maybe Dr. Teng had mentioned it to him. We talked turns and ski areas. I gave him my card with the photo of me from the freestyling days, and information about my autobiography.

"Read that. You will learn a lot. Not only about skiing but about life."

"Thanks I will get it."

"My website is on the back or get it on Amazon." I continued, "All seems to be working well. Call Dr. Teng and ask him if I can go home. I am peeing more and retaining less. I'm good to go."

"I'll call him. Only he can make the decision."

"Thanks."

He found Dr. Teng in another hospital. When he was told the results, he said I could go home.

"He agreed. I will tell them to get your paperwork ready."

"Thanks for calling him. Everyone here has been exceptional. I appreciate it. Be sure to get the book."

Twenty minutes later, I was on my way home.

Saturday, 18 November 2017 and onwards.

Over the next days and weeks, there were no unexpected surprises. Everything that I was told or read had happened. There was some intermittent bleeding with burning to various degrees. I bought a powder called Ural that, when mixed with water, neutralizes the acidity and reduces the stinging and the need to stand on tiptoe. Otherwise taking Ibuprofen helped. I felt the effects of the anesthetic drugs, which made me tired and slightly dizzy. I was told to take a mega B complex, a mixture of many of the B vitamins, and that cleared up those symptoms in one day. I have had no other side effects. The stream has improved and is often like the old days where the foam comes over the bowl! Okay, a slight exaggeration.

March 2018

Everything is working, as it should, thanks to Dr. Teng. I cannot stress enough the importance of having a second opinion and finding the best doctor. It can save your life and a lot of pain.

Now, there is an ongoing fight with Garfield Hospital because they refused to provide a truthful report and subsequently I'm not able to claim travel insurance. I have told them a lawsuit is the next step. They made an offer that I refused, which only told me that they realize they are guilty of malpractice. I have told them what I want and if not, the lawsuit proceeds. I am waiting the result.

October 2018

It has been just over a year since this adventure or misadventure began. Garfield Hospital has steadfastly refused to send a truthful report of the circumstances and I have not been able to involve my insurance.

After months of back and forth, offers and counteroffers, a settlement was reached. Garfield without any admission of wrongdoing agreed to pay all outstanding bills as well as a sum to me for 'pain and suffering'. To end the episode, I signed a non-disclosure statement on the amount of the financial settlement.

What, if anything, have I learned from all of this?

You never think about having to urinate until you can't.

To all the gents, if at any time your 'flow' changes see your doctor without delay or suffer the consequences. If you have problems with passing water, even a stream that is weak at times, check it out early and avoid a history like the one you have read here. Know your body, find a good doctor that you have confidence in, and call on Dr. Google when you have a question.

If I had done any of these, the six-hour ride would never have been as much fun as anticipated!

Men are notorious for avoiding the obvious when it comes to their bodies. I am the perfect example of this and been lucky to not have had medical problems before. Now, I will still avoid running to a doctor. However, I will listen more closely as age brings about changes to the way my body performs and feels. I have a lot to accomplish. I have no fear of dying but fear of not doing all I plan to do before that time.

Life is short. Do it today.

jk

Top Ten Takeaways

1. The male prostate increases in size at puberty and continues to grow, doubling in size between ages 21 – 50, and doubling again by 80 years of age.

2. Benign Prostatic Hyperplasia (BPH) refers a prostate gland that has increased in size of without malignancy present.

3. Some men don't have any problems even though their prostate has enlarged.

4. Bladder Outlet Obstruction is the most common problem caused by an enlarged prostate in that it surrounds and narrows the top part of the urethra and affects the flow of urine. See your doctor if you have any obstructive symptoms before a total block causes emergency treatment.

5. From the age of 50, all men should have regular prostate checks and discussions with their doctor and, if necessary, their urologists. This means a Digital Rectum Exam (DRE) from a male or female doctor.

6. If you have a family history of prostate cancer, these checks should start earlier.

7. Prostate Specific Antigen (PSA) results on their own do not indicate prostate cancer. Fluctuations over time indicate that cells are changing and further investigation may be necessary.

8. Prostate health can be strengthened by maintaining a healthy weight with a good diet, plenty of exercise and reduced stress to insure your immune system is not compromised.

9. Don't be afraid to seek a second medical opinion. Plenty of information is also available on the internet. Listening to the experiences of friends and relatives is also helpful.

10. Be sure you trust your doctor and fully understand all the issues. If you don't, ask questions.

TALL TALES TWO

Bill's Story

Originally My Story by William Van Atten

When I turned fifty, as part of my annual physical, my doctor ordered a PSA (Prostate Specific Antigen) test for the first time. As many of you probably know, this is a blood test for possible prostate cancer, the second leading cause of death in men.

About a week after the test was administered, I received a call from my doctor advising that the test result was positive. What a surprise.

All I could say was, "What do I do now?

The doctor's answer was that many times this test gives a 'false positive' so we wait three months and do the test again.

Well, I had to live for those three months not knowing if I had cancer or not. What a time of anxiety.

When they did the test again, I saw my doctor face-to-face for the results. He told me my second test had come out fine so I was one of the ones who got a 'false positive' result and "sorry you had to wait three months to find out." What a relief that was, but it was hell waiting the three months to find out.

Soon after, I got a new job in New York City and had to relocate from Massachusetts. This meant a change of doctors. When I found a new one and had my annual exam, I asked about a PSA test. He said he didn't believe in them because of all the false positives. He believed in the good old finger exam. After my prior experience, I agreed with him, so no more PSA tests. Ten years passed and I lived fine without any PSA tests.

One of my passions was ski racing and I was able to compete in Masters racing for years. While perhaps a little older and slower, I felt like I was an Olympic racer even though the racecourses were the same, challenging courses that you would get at college level.

One of the competitions I participated in was the Eastern Regional Masters Championships. While running a Super G course, an event that is very close to a Downhill course except there are a few gates to maneuver through, I had a terrific crash leaving me with multiple injuries. I had a ruptured spleen, a torn rotator cuff, and a fractured diaphragm, which left part of my stomach in my chest cavity (not good for the digestion).

Each of these injuries required surgery but the ruptured spleen required emergency surgery as I was bleeding out internally. This was done in the ER. The rotator cuff was operated on about four weeks later as they wanted to space the surgeries a month apart because of my age as a senior citizen. These first two surgeries went fine.

Then came the diaphragm surgery. Firstly, this required going into the abdomen, pulling the stomach down and attaching it. Secondly, the diaphragm itself had to be sown back together. When I woke up, the surgeon told me everything went well except for one problem they'd encountered. She asked me when I last had a PSA test. I told her it was about ten years ago because my General Practitioner didn't believe in them.

"Well," she said, "we could not get a catheter inserted after we put you under and had to call the urologist to do the insertion. He had to use a small hammer device to do it so if you experience some bleeding that is the cause but you need to get a PSA test immediately."

This scared me so I scheduled one as soon as I was released from the hospital starting me on a long road of prostate cancer discovery and treatment.

I had the PSA test done and the results came back as elevated. The urologist then told me to come back in a month to do the test again so we could be sure we didn't have a false positive. I nervously waited the month and had the test again. It came out elevated again. The doctor then said he had to do the next level of test (code for more expensive and not covered by insurance unless you have two PSA tests first). This entailed milking the prostate and collecting a sample of the milk. Not pleasant unless you like that sort of thing. The sample was sent off and the result a week later was positive.

♂

So I had the big "C." Now what to do about it.

I went back to the urologist for a consultation. He said that now we had to do a biopsy to see how extensive the cancer was. He explained that they divide the prostate into quadrants and take two biopsy samples from each. This meant eight samples.

I said, "Okay, here we go."

The samples are taken by inserting a device up the rectum. Simply stated, they shoot a little arrow into the prostate to get the sample. The doctor put me in position.

Whoosh went the first shot and I almost went off the table.

He didn't tell me in advance that it was going to hurt. Wow, and now I knew with ONLY seven more to go! I left his office that day walking very gingerly.

Back to the doctor for the biopsy results. He told me the cancer was only in two quadrants so this is considered early stage. I had a number of options that he outlined as follows:

- Wait and see. I was on the cusp of old age where I might die of something else before the cancer developed.

- Radiation directed at the cancerous part of the prostate with all kinds of side effects.

- Complete removal of the prostate surgically either by hand or robotically.

- Little radioactive beads placed into the affected part of the prostate to kill the cancer cells.

The urologist said if he removed the prostate completely, I would be a eunuch. Well, this needed some reflection and research. I am an analytical type so off I went with my head spinning. The first thing I did, of course, was Google the life out of my computer. There is a lot of information there. It turns out that prostate cancer is the second leading cause of death in men so this had to be treated very seriously.

Then there is family history. I remember that my grandfather died of prostate cancer. This was back in the sixties. He had radiation treatments but then it spread into his bones. Near the end, he could not be touched as his bones were disintegrating. It was a terrible and painful way to go.

I started talking to friends my age and found that a lot of them had dealt with prostate cancer. All I had to do was ask and a plethora of information poured out. I didn't realize how pervasive it was. Most of them were ski instructors like myself and led very active lives. One just had it completely removed. He could never get it up again and complained that he had to wear diapers for a year. Another had radiation and told me he has never been the same. Ditto, no sexual activity possible.

My thoughts were that it is better to be alive and limp than dead with a hard-on. I didn't like the wait-and-see scenario. Too many unknowns. Just knowing that prostate cancer metastasizes into the bones and works its way throughout your skeleton, the pictures of bone cancer on Google convinced me that I was not going to wait.

My studies then centered around robotic surgery as the best way to go. It was referred to as the 'Gold Standard' in prostate surgery. It had the reputation for getting all the cancer cleanly so it did not return. You not only want robotic surgery but you want the most skilled surgeon. I found that there was a correlation between skill and the number of surgeries performed. It made sense that the more practice you have, the better you get. I zeroed in on a surgeon at a New York City teaching hospital who had done about 2,500 prostate removals with a robot. He became my guy.

I saw him several times and scheduled my surgery. It's a four-hour procedure. On the appointed day, they prepped me and then wheeled me into the operating room. There were two anesthesiologists, which made me feel good after seeing what happened to Michael Jackson. I asked why my surgeon wasn't there too. Everyone laughed and said he was in a different room to control the robot. I could see two huge robotic arms being positioned next to me and then I was out.

♂

I woke up in the recovery room six hours later. When they eventually wheeled me up to my room, I was told I had to get up and walk. I thought the nurse was joking but she was serious. You have to work off the anesthesia. Although my legs were shaking and I was attached to an IV and a catheter, I managed a few laps down the hall and back. By this time it was 10:00 pm and they finally let me get some sleep. Of course, they wake you up every few hours for a vital-signs check.

The next morning the surgeon came in and told me everything had gone well. There were no signs that the cancer had spread. Then with a smile, he told me he was able to save my nerve bundle. He seemed to make a big deal about it but I had no clue as to what he was talking about. He said that this is possible only with the precision of robotic surgery. I was still in a groggy state so did not know what questions to ask him.

After he left, I was able to get out my iPad and Google 'nerve bundle'. OMG! These are the nerves, which control erections. I was still a male capable of performing. Something I didn't think would be possible. How glad was I that I chose robotic surgery. I didn't even catch this in my research and thought my sex life would be all over after the operation.

I was discharged that afternoon. They sure don't keep you in the hospital very long these days. A four-hour surgery and they kick you out the next day with a large catheter bag and an abdomen drain.

I had to wear the bag and drain for two weeks, then go back to see the doctor. They took out the big catheter and drain bag; and gave me a smaller catheter and bag. Then they fitted me out with disposable diapers that I needed to wear after complete removal of the catheters. Back to diapers felt embarrassing. So this is one of the reasons why every pharmacy has a half an aisle of disposable diapers! They also gave me a three-month prescription for Cialis to use daily to stimulate the blood flow around my lower abdomen.

Then it was come back in another month to check my PSA level. When I went back, the doctor said that the healing process would take about one year so don't expect to have a lot of sexual activity. He added that if I liked, they could give me a prescription for a hormone and chemical mix that is very effective for producing an erection but it had to be injected directly into the penis.

After all the pain I had endured, I said I would like to try it. They had me meet with a male nurse (not a beautiful female nurse) who showed me how to administer the injection. They then loaded up a syringe and told me to give it a go. I injected a small amount and, voila, I had an erection within five minutes. They called in the prescription, which had to be mixed and sent refrigerated to my home. I left the doctor's office thinking life was not so bad.

When my Trimix prescription arrived, I thought I would give it a try. I had been warned by the nurse to be very careful about the dosage. Too much could produce an erection lasting more than four hours called a priapism, meaning a persistent and painful erection of the penis. Four hours! In my dreams, I thought. My wife was not thrilled with my new virility as she had gone through menopause and complained of a dry vagina. It was only much later that I found out it wasn't dry but rather she was having fun with others behind my back. Anyway, that is a whole other story.

A few months after getting my Trimix, I gave myself too much of a dose. After four or five hours, in the middle of the night, I went to the hospital by myself to see how fast I could have this dealt with. At the ER, the nurse asked me what my problem was. As there were dozens of other people in the waiting room, in a low voice, I told her I had a priapism.

She said, "What is that?"

She didn't know what I was talking about so I then had to explain that I have an erection that has lasted more than four hours. That she understood and gave me a priority admittance.

They wheeled me on a gurney and put me into an examination room with another person. I was told that they had to get the on-call urologist to do the procedure needed. The man in the room with me said they thought he'd had a heart attack and he had been waiting there for fifteen hours.

A resident doctor came in. He did something to me that just made me bleed constantly. I could see the sheet turning red beneath me. The man next to me said he was going to sue the hospital. How could anyone with a heart attack be left waiting for fifteen hours for treatment? Was I going to bleed out?

Finally, the urologist arrived and wheeled me into a room by myself. Sadly, I saw they had wheeled another person out into the aisle to make room for me. The urologist said that their new residents had just started last week and would I mind if they watched the procedure. I was half out of my mind by then and said sure.

In came about a dozen newly minted doctors to gaze at my throbbing erection. And half of them were women. So the doctor did the procedure while fielding questions from the observing residents. Soon all the blood was drained out and I felt much better.

My story is just about over except for a few more things. Over time, I found that I not only had an erection but also had a climax with nothing coming out. Then I started to be multi-orgasmic just like a female. I would have one orgasm after another with only a minute or two between each. Wow, this made me happy as well as my partner. So for all the trauma I went through due to the cancer, there was a happy ending.

I sincerely hope that men reading this will be able to make more informed decisions about any potential prostate cancer. Get a PSA test and digital exam every year if you are over fifty, no matter what your doctor says. I was lucky to have discovered the cancer early due to an accident. That was true luck.

♂♂♂♂♂

George

George Myros looked at himself in the mirror. The Hollywood lights above the mirror reflected a perfect image. *"Not bad for fifty-nine,"* he thought. He carefully stroked his moustache and straightened his shirt collar. One more look and he was ready. George was as prepared as could be to step into the murky world of online dating.

Martha Myros had died suddenly only a month after being diagnosed with cervical cancer. They had found it too late. George and his family grieved her passing. The two children, John and his sister Lena, two years younger, went back to their homes and families in other parts of the country, a few days after Martha was in her final resting place. They assured their father they were there for him if there was anything he needed. George convinced them he would be okay and although he would miss his wife of thirty-six years, he would spend time with the friends he had and his hobbies, playing golf and following many other sports.

For all his bravado, George hadn't quite realized that the house would feel so empty and how alone he would be. It was a large old house with four bedrooms, a spacious kitchen, and a back deck, which was used more as a living room than the living area in the front of the house. After a few months of sitting around and feeling sorry for himself, he'd had enough. Nothing was going to bring Martha back and doing nothing wasn't any way to live.

He decided to modernize the house. Out went the furniture except for what had been in the kid's bedrooms. A van belonging to an organization working with the homeless hauled it all away, including the kitchen appliances. Even the carpets were torn up and the light fittings removed. George wanted a fresh, new environment with few memories reflecting what had been. This had been taken away from him, not by choice, and no amount of wanting was ever going to change that.

He consulted with a few interior decorators before hiring Decon Weber & Co. He told them his ideas. They listened and suggested. Decisions were made and the negotiations on the price began in earnest. George worked for himself as a successful buyer's agent for those seeking a new or used car at a very good price. He used his skills on Decon Weber. The outcome was that it would take more than three weeks for the revamping of the house to be completed and for much less than he anticipated paying.

George rented a unit near the beach about 30 miles away. This enabled him to inspect the work but not be living in the midst of it. The family SUV was sold and he now drove an Infinity coupe in red. It looked as if it was moving when it stood still.

Emerging as the new George, and not being the type to do things by halves, George also started the process of changing how he dressed. More stylish clothing, mod, but not over the top for his age. Slacks and white shirts went out, replaced by polos and jeans. Black shoes were boxed up and given away. His closet now had a variety of Nike, New Balance, Sketchers and Clarks. Sitting on the beach, George was working on tanning his six-foot, 183-pound frame. Without his wife, his life changed drastically. To cope, he was continuing the process.

After much soul-searching, George decided he could now adjust and not have any problems living alone. Having the freedom to do what he wanted, when he wanted, appealed to him. Cooking was something he enjoyed so he wasn't concerned about food.

Sex? Sex was the thing on his mind for which he would have to find a solution. This was not as easy as revamping a house or having a wardrobe makeover. He had been out of the dating game for many years. Things had changed even when his children were going through it. Did he have the skills required in today's world? Where does he start? Pickup bars were not his thing. Hookers? No challenge there. Join up with a church group. Not likely. It was more of a conundrum that would need further thought.

WOW!

That was the only word that came to mind when George walked through his renovated home. Room by room, it was far better than he had anticipated. Sure, it had cost more than the agreed amount but what the hell was money for if not to be spent. He had spent years with Martha saying they did not need this, the old one was good enough, or we can wait until it stops working. Those days were over.

The new TV screen was three times bigger than the old one. The sofa was leather, the down lights were on dimmers, and the kitchen appliances were state-of-the-art modern. The whole house smelled new. It felt good and suited the future that George now envisaged. Lying on his new bed catching sight of himself in the mirrored closet doors was so far removed from the bedroom he had known for so many years.

An island bench was the center of the new kitchen. Within arm's reach was a new capsule coffee machine, which George thought made the best coffee that he had ever tasted and it was in his house. Gone was the tin-tasting percolator. George sat on a stool in shorts, no shirt or shoes, reading the news on a new slim-line laptop. He thought he heard the doorbell but was not sure with Tommy James shouting out 'Mony Mony' through the music system wired into every room.

"Lord Jesus, what has happened to the house," shouted Doris over the music.

George looked up to see his sister-in-law standing there holding an aluminum-foil-covered dish.

"Alexa. Stop," George said to the black speaker post sitting near the coffee machine. The room went quiet.

Doris stood with her mouth open, aghast at what she saw.

"Where are all the family photos that were on the walls?"

"In here," said George pointing to his head.

"Have you lost control of your senses since my sister died? She would turn over in her grave if she saw this house. I am so happy she is spared the misery. Look at you. No shirt and its midday. You can ask for help you know. We are here for you."

"Martha is gone. Life goes on. I needed a change. A new start. I like it."

"What have you done with all the beautiful furniture and antiques? This place looks like a waiting room in a brothel. I have never seen one but it would look like this I'm sure," Doris spoke loudly with disgust in her voice.

George stared at her and as he did, he mentally undressed her. Her black dress slipped away and her large brassiere revealed one breast larger than the other with the nipples on both pointing towards her shoes. The dress dropped further and then the bloomers. A forest as thick as any Amazon thicket ranged from her belly button to half way to her knees. George quickly shook his head erasing the vision from his mind.

"Alexa, play a song with jungle in the title."

The hard rock sound of 'Welcome to the Jungle' by Guns & Roses filled the house. A smile crossed George's face. How appropriate he thought.

"George, what is that noise and where did it come from? I am so upset I am not leaving the food I brought for you. You have disgraced my sister's memory." Doris turned and stomped out of the house.

"That went well," thought George. *"I think she liked the house!"*

"Alexa play the Eagles," and the music suddenly changed to 'Desperado'.

George popped another capsule into the machine and waited for the coffee to fill his cup. "*Am I a desperado? I have been a good husband all my life. Yes a few times, no sometimes, I strayed but my excuse was valid. Martha thought sex was to procreate and not for fun. It was not her fault. Her upbringing and family. I could never change her. I hoped for years that she would enjoy sex. She never did. She accommodated me but it wasn't enough. I wanted to feel I excited her like Slutty Sandra, the girl from the neighborhood, who had it off with anyone, including me. Now she was always excited and wet like a river.*"

The coffee relaxed George and his mind wandered back many years. "*I was always happy with Martha. She was a terrific mother. I truly loved her. I asked her to go with me on those trips but she never would. Car conventions in Detroit and Vegas were part of my job to keep abreast of the changes in the industry. It was not all work. There was some play that started innocently enough at a party and progressed to my room with the wife of an executive who was more sex starved than I was. Once that door was opened, there was no way to close it. I only played around when out of town. I never brought it home with me. I kept it in another world where I was another person. No one was hurt.*" George got up and put the cup in the sink. *"I won't hurt Martha now. I don't have to answer to Doris or anyone."*

The sun burned into George's chest. It felt good, charging him up and tanning his skin. Two women walked by him without noticing him at all. *"Am I invisible?"* he thought. There was a day when women noticed him, smiled and often said hello. Now, whether on the beach or in the supermarket, George was a ghost. Could he remedy this or was there no answer other than accept that it was the scourge of old age?

The beach was becoming crowded. George picked up his towel, put on his shorts and t-shirt before walking to the nearest café. He took a seat where he could watch tourists and locals wandering by. Thin bodies, fat ones, and all sorts in between. Big tits, small breasts, and those hardly discernable competed for attention with long hair, short cuts, tattoos, piercings, and those walking dogs. The circus before his eyes made it difficult to figure out which kind of woman would attract him. Truthfully, he had no idea except if they said yes.

While sitting on his newly refurbished deck watching a baseball game on the wall-mounted TV mounted, an advertisement came on showing a happy smiling couple running along a beach. The text said, 'Where friendship becomes love. Fusion. Online dating with lasting results.' After the game finished, George thought about the ad.

"Online dating. Sitting at home and choosing who you want to meet makes sense." He went into the house to get his laptop and investigate the possibilities.

George opened the window to the chaotic world of online dating. Besides someone's top ten sites, RSVP, Zoosk, Elite Singles, Match, eHarmony, Silver Singles, Naughty Date, Tinder, be2, and Plenty Of Fish, there are specialty sites such as, Christian Mingle, Senior People Meet, Black People Meet, Gay Match Maker, among countless others.

If that wasn't enough, there are the sites bordering on the ridiculous: Purrsonals.com for cat lovers, Amish-online-dating, Clown Dating, Ugly Schmucks, Farmers Only, Mullet Passions, (the hairstyle not the fish), Diaper Mates, and Sugar Daddies.

George got up from his computer and headed to the fridge for a beer. *"This may take a lot longer than I thought. There is something for everyone, like in a grocery store. Choose a body with the attributes you desire instead of a breakfast food with nuts, fruits or gluten free."* While sipping his beer, George sat in front of the screen and brought up RSVP, one of the top ten and most popular.

He navigated his way around, learning that if you actually wanted to contact someone you had to buy stamps. Before this, you had to establish a profile providing some personal information as well as describing yourself. Adding a photo was optional but recommended to attract more interest.

Most of the sites he visited worked in much the same way. Some were completely free. Relating free to the business sense that you usually get what you paid for, he avoided the free sites and decided to put his profile up on three sites. RSVP, eHarmony, and Tinder.

In his mind, based on what he read and saw, RSVP was finding a date, eHarmony was looking for the life-long partner and Tinder was sex only, if that was the goal. George was unsure what he was actually looking for so choosing these three seemed to cover all bases. Now to work on his profile.

He read many profiles getting an idea of what people wrote. It was not long before he understood the world was full of beautiful people who spent most of their time either walking on the beach or in the bush. All others were at either the gym or a sporting event.

He matched the photos to what the individuals had written. He didn't have to be a detective to determine that many of the walkers and gym-goers had made more than one detour to the fridge or pantry. Photos may not lie but he suspected people did.

After looking at profiles without photos, he figured he would have to provide a photo with his profile to draw attention to it. George looked through photos on his computer and found one with his wife at a cocktail party. He expertly cropped the photo so only a picture of him smiling remained. *"That will work,"* he thought.

Writing a profile was far more difficult. To start, he had to come up with a name to use on the sites and a catchy headline. There were many false starts before he decided to go with basic information. Age, height and his likes, travel, dining, and conversation. He added he was widowed and had no children at home. There was no mention of beach walking in the moonlight.

He added his profile to the three sites. Now all he had to do was wait for the replies. In the meantime, he would play a round or two of golf.

Two days later, to his surprise, George had over twenty replies to his profile. He drank a beer while considering each one. George knew that his tastes went to women with what he considered a 'normal' body. Obese was not his thing nor was too thin. Huge tits were like new toys, after you played with them a few times they were old toys. Nothing exaggerated would be fine for him as long as there was conversation and a few laughs.

George selected two women. One on RSVP named Silvia and the other on eHarmony. Silvia stated she was forty-five, divorced, and liked to travel. Her photo appealed to him. He asked to meet her in a café. The idea excited him.

Betty was a divorcee looking for a relationship. She had ideas of her perfect man, which she said she would explain in due time. George liked her photo. Big smile, short blondish hair, and something in her face attracted him but he could not say what. He also asked to meet with her.

Some of the others, he wanted to chat with and keep them in mind in case Silvia and Betty didn't work out.

Later in the day, he had a message from Betty asking three questions. What was his religion? Did he contribute to charities, and what was his idea of a good meal? George thought these were strange questions. Without online experience, he went along with the demand, answering that he had let go of his religious beliefs, that he contributed to the needy and that he liked Thai food.

A short time later, he received a reply from Betty. More questions. How important is family to you? Do you own your own home? Do you agree a close friendship is very important before any intimacy? George reread the questions. Then he laughed. I am not interested in any of this. I want to meet and have a chat. He asked to meet and discuss her topics in person.

Her answer was swift and direct. "I do not meet until I am sure of who I am meeting with. eHarmony is excellent in protecting its users until such a time they both agree to meet. You have not answered my questions."

"The hell with this. I don't need an interrogation. I'm only looking for some fun. I'll cancel eHarmony," was George's reaction. He went to the website to cancel. After an hour of trying, he found there was no way he could figure out how to cancel. There was always some message produced to hinder that option. George then had a better idea. He would change his profile. He went to the profile bar and clicked Edit.

Occupation: Pimp

Looking for: Women free to work part-time. Housewives accepted.

Body type: Big to huge tits

Serious replies only

George hit the save button.

Thirty minutes later George was banned from the site for life. With that success, his thoughts now turned to Silvia as she had agreed to meet.

Silvia was a nice person. She looked like her photo and as far as George could tell was about the age she had indicated. They seemed to have things in common except Silvia smoked. Not one, but one after another. George could not abide being around smokers and he sure as hell had no intention of kissing one. After coffee, he told Silvia he would call. Both knew he would not.

Not one to be discouraged, George set about changing his profile. He now included:

- Non-smokers only
- Aged 45 - 55
- No children living at home
- Education – professional
- Within 25 miles
- Willing to meet

George examined what he'd added. He thought that should eliminate a few. He went back and looked over the other responses without finding anyone who caught his attention. I will wait and see what happens once the women out there have a chance to read my updated profile.

The 10:00 am meeting was in a coffee shop. She had told him on the phone that she would be wearing a blue jacket. George got there early and selected a table where he had a clear view of everyone entering. He spotted her from a distance. The blue jacket moved through the café towards his table. She stopped abruptly and put out her hand.

"George? You look like your photo. Carol. Nice to meet you. I'll have café latte, please."

In one motion, George stood, shook her hand and summoned the waitress, as he watched her sit down. She was seventy and that was being kind. He listened with one ear as she explained how she had taken the bus to get there on time, but his head was thinking of ways to bail out in a polite manner.

The coffee arrived. Carol drank it and talked at the same time with dribble leaking from the corner of her mouth. Now it was about her cat and the talking continued non-stop.

"Excuse me. My phone is vibrating. It's my office. Give me a minute please."

George moved away from the table towards the door. He spoke into the phone while making hand gestures and returned to the table.

"Carol I am very sorry. An emergency at the office. I have to leave. Enjoy the coffee."

He left a $10 bill on the table and made haste to the door. As he drove he thought. *"Rule number one of online dating: PEOPLE LIE."*

The 5:00 pm meeting, as George now understood, was not a meeting but more of an interview. Interview was a word that described the encounter far more clearly than a meeting. The spot he had picked was an upmarket wine bar with outside seating. Flo, as she called herself was blond in her photo. Her profile read 'age 48, 5' 8 tall'. What had interested George was the line, 'I am interested in self-understanding through experiences.' He had no idea what she meant. It sounded like more fun than bushwalking.

Wearing a black polo with black jeans, George parked across from the bar. Walking towards the outside tables, he could see her sitting there sipping a glass of wine He looked at his watch. 5:05. Not very late. Flo was every bit as attractive as her photo. She wore a dark dress with a low-cut front. Her body was athletic, her smile inviting.

After the introductions, George ordered two glasses of house champagne

"George, have you met many women online?"

Taken by surprise by the direct question, George answered, "I am new to this. I have met a couple. They were not my type or perhaps I was not theirs."

"What is your type, George?"

George observed her as she talked. Maybe she was a hooker or maybe she was just in a hurry to get the important interview questions out of the way so as not to waste her time.

"Now if I knew what that was, I would have advertised for exactly that in my profile. Until I know, I will settle for someone who makes me laugh while enjoying some time together. What about you?"

"George, I don't think I'm your type."

"How would you know that in five minutes?"

"Because George, you are a nice man. I am not as I seem. I am into BDSM and I'm quite sure you have no idea what I am talking about." Flo watched George with a questioning face.

Before George could answer, Flo explained.

"Bondage and discipline, dominance and submission, and sadism and masochism. Sounds like quite a handful. Pretty far outside the ordinary, isn't it? But, it isn't as extraordinary as you might think. Many women are into various facets and degrees of this, me included."

She could see George had a stunned look on his face.

"You are about to ask me a hundred questions. If you want to know more, go online where there are plenty of sites to inform you. It was nice to meet you. Thanks for the champagne."

Flo was up and gone before George could protest. He ordered another champagne. "*What just happened,*" he thought. She was right. He had questions he wanted to ask. The image of her body naked, tied up, or handcuffed with a studded dog collar around her neck aroused him. What happened then? Did someone beat her or just tease her? George had no idea. He drained his champagne. She was right. Flo was not his type. There was so much to learn in this online dating game.

The next week George had arranged four different 'interviews'. For one, he had traveled further than he wanted but was attracted to the photo and her profile. Charlotte was cute and bubbly. George felt at ease with her immediately. They were at a café where they ordered lunch and talked effortlessly.

"I haven't had much chance to travel in the past few years. I'm going to remedy this and take a few trips in the next couple of months. Naturally it would be more fun to have someone accompany me."

"I have never been out of the State. I have never been on a plane and never intend to. I am happy here and have no desire to move at all."

George could not believe what he heard. "You don't want to see other things and visit places you have heard about?"

"No, not at all. I have no interest in it."

"Well Charlotte, I guess we would be a bad match. I want to travel and not alone. This will not work out. Thanks for meeting with me."

Where before George worried about being polite and perhaps hurting someone's feelings, he was now quick to bail out when he understood the person was not for him.

Meetings took a lot of time. It was important to put your time to good use and not waste it in situations that were going nowhere. A case in point was where George made plans to meet a woman in an outdoor café. They arranged that he would be wearing a blue shirt and she a green sweater. George wore a white shirt and spotted the woman in green from afar. As he closed in, he realized she was far older and not in the least as she was represented in her photo and profile. George did an about-turn and left the area.

Did his behavior trouble him? Yes. Luckily, George was a fast learner, especially with learning opportunities emerging with each meeting. People lie about their age and many things, photos are years out of date, they have children when they say they don't, they are divorced when still married, and so on.

Online dating is a cutthroat affair. If you are too nice, you will be hurt. If you treat it as a business interview, you may survive. Another two meetings were a quick drink, a few words with 'you are not my type' and 'goodbye'. More lessons learned.

In six weeks of online dating, got George laid once. She was short with large breasts. Her manner was direct as they drank a glass of wine.

"Look, you want to get laid and so do I. I am not into long conversations and beating around the bush. It's in the bush if you get my meaning. Let's go to your place."

George hesitated with his answer, as he was wary that she might want to case his house for a later visit to rob anything of value. She was well dressed but that meant very little. He was horny, which led to thinking with his dick instead of his head.

"Follow me."

"Okay. I have about an hour and a half before I have to get the kids from school. Life can be hell for a single mother. You have to take your pleasure when you can. Lead the way."

The woman, who decided it was unimportant for George to know her name, followed him in a late-model station wagon. Still being suspicious, George noted the number plate and wrote it down. If she came back for the flat screen TV, maybe he could find her.

Driving towards his house, he felt somewhat apprehensive. It was the first time he would have sex in his home with someone other than his wife. It was then that his dick spoke, reminding him that it had to happen eventually; better now than tomorrow; a bird in hand; and all the other clichés. George drove on.

Two hours later George sat on the back deck with a beer, smiling. He fingered the embossed card as he read and reread the name, Shirley Ganner, Media Associates as he recalled her words before she left his house.

"You're a good fuck George. Anytime you want another session, give me a call."

Replaying the action in his mind he realized he had not done all that much except follow orders. Shirley gave the directions. He followed. Everyone was satisfied. There weren't any worries that she would revisit for the TV but it was highly likely she would make another appearance.

Next came Rita. What a contrast in personality to Shirley. Rita had reluctantly agreed to meet George in the food court of a shopping center at noon saying it was a safe place to meet someone for the first time.

George gave her the once over as he took a seat at the table with her. Pleasant enough to look at, body on the slim side but dressed in clothing that better suited someone quite a few years older.

"You look like your photo. So far so good. Let's get right into it." Rita said as she pulled a yellow legal pad from her oversized handbag. "You stated that you are fifty-nine. Is that correct?"

"Yes it is," answered George, silently amused at the proceedings.

"You have a full time job?" Seeing him nod his head she said, "Okay."

"You own your own home? You have no children living with you? Friendship is of value to you?"

The questions kept coming. George politely butted in and asked, "What is your position on sex?"

Rita stared at George.

"I'm sorry. I didn't mean what position you might enjoy. I meant to say, do you think sex is important in a relationship?"

In a stern voice Rita replied, "Let me tell you this. My husband and I courted for more than six months before the subject came up. Friendship is the most important thing in any relationship. We were soul mates to the day he died. Friendship first. Sex takes care of itself when there is friendship and as you get older it becomes less and less, if at all important."

"I disagree with you. Sex, to me, is important. It grows friendship. It may not be the same as a teenager out behind the barn, but in bed it never wanes much at any age."

"You are just like the rest. Sex is all that is on your mind. You are a disappointment to me, George or whatever you name is. I will say goodbye now."

George watched her walk away. "*I handled that quite well*," he thought. He remembered that in many of his past meetings the word friendship came up far more often than the topic of sex. "*The majority seem to be lacking in friends where as I miss sex. Back to the computer to try again.*"

Every day George was overwhelmed with the number of responses he received. It was impossible to answer them all and very time-consuming sorting through them to see who would be good to connect with. Even with careful culling, most meetings, while improving his education, proved little more than conversation.

Sandra was a schoolteacher. Her profile was similar to his with a photo showing an attractive woman. George messaged her, which led to talking to her on the phone. She invited him to her house for a late-afternoon tea. That was the first time he had had such an invite. This had George excited. Maybe at last he was about to meet someone who he would want to meet again.

The townhouse was in a gated community. George buzzed the number as instructed and the gates opened. The houses were clearly numbered making it easy to find the one where Sandra was waiting by the door.

"Welcome. Come in. You look like your photo which is a welcome surprise."

"Nice to be invited. Thank you."

George stepped into a spacious living area carefully decorated in a feminine style.

"Please have a seat while I get you a coffee, or would you like tea?"

"Coffee please. I read that you are a teacher. What grade?"

"Sixth. I'll answer all your questions in a minute. Let me get the drinks."

Sandra returned with coffee as well as a tray of freshly baked little cakes. George had one and asked for another.

"These are delicious. I presume you made them."

"I did. I like to cook when I have the time."

The conversation flowed with ease. It was like they were old friends. Both felt comfortable as the time flew by.

"I hate to end this when it has been so much fun but I have a few hours of papers to correct. We will have to meet again."

"I would like that," said George standing to leave. "Next time it will be my treat."

"Next time you can come here and I will cook you dinner. I would enjoy that and after dinner, if we get along, we can have more fun. Come with me."

George followed her into a large bedroom with a king-sized bed. Sandra stopped in front of a chest of drawers. She opened the middle of three and peeled back a cover.

"Look at this. I told you we could be in for a lot of fun."

George's mouth dropped open and his eyes widened. Before him in the drawer, precisely laid out, were two dildos, one larger than the other, a strap-on belt with huge cock, a two-headed dildo at least eighteen inches long, and a selection of vibrators in assorted sizes, shapes, and colors.

"My friends that I like to share with my special guests! I said we could have fun after dinner," Sandra said with a confident smile.

George, a man not usually lost for words, was speechless. Finally, he managed, "That is quite a collection."

"When I decide, I make it memorable. My friends can be your friends too."

"I am sure you do." George turned away and walked from the bedroom.

In the living area, he turned and thanked her once again. Sandra kissed him on the cheek and whispered, "Call me when you want to come for dinner."

George nodded and left. Once out of the gates he sped away towards his home. He grinned and grimaced at the same time as his mind pictured what might happen if he was to decide to become friends with Sandra's friends.

After three months very little had changed. While meeting with many more women who were nice enough, they didn't measure up to what George was looking for. He was aware that in some cases he was the one who fell below expectations.

Some of his golf friends tried to fix him up with friends of their wives. That was not going to happen. In George's mind that would be like a substitute for his deceased wife. The old saying that there is someone for everyone was losing credence. Seek and you shall find made more sense.

George sat in front of his computer and reviewed his profile. Something about this online dating bothered him. An informative profile and up-to-date photo got results. Too many, in fact. It was like the shotgun approach to hitting a flock of birds of which almost all were undesirable. *"What if I wrote a profile that will do the opposite. Scare the majority of the birds away leaving only the ones who will be drawn by the precise wording."* The more he considered it, the more George liked the idea.

Excited by how clever this new slant would be, he set to work rewriting his profile. A few hours and a few beers later, the profile with new headline, was ready to post, designed to generate far fewer responses. Any woman who did reply would in line with the mentality he was hoping to find.

His new profile now included the following:

TAKE THE TEST

- Walk on the beach or fly in a hot air balloon?
- Bushwalk or ride in a high-speed rally car?
- Sit and watch a DVD or cuddle up and become a star?

Any wrong answer, push the escape button now.

I am private, confident, educated, & experienced.

Call me shallow because I am when it comes to what attracts me. No attraction, no hope. Please, no overweight bodies!!

I'M LOOKING FOR:

A woman who seeks an experienced mature gentleman, educated, exciting, and adventurous. In order not to waste my time or yours, I prefer a slim body, but an open-mind or a certain look can be enough. SEXUAL COMPATABILITY before friendship. Willing to meet for dating or a relationship.

Apart from the direct statements regarding body type, there was nothing too unusual in the profile except one sentence that George knew would be the deciding factor in reducing the many responses to a very few.

'Sexual compatibility before friendship.'

Many going online are lonely and seeking friendship more than sex. They tolerate and may even enjoy sex as part of the bargain but don't consider it important. George was not lonely nor did he need any more friends.

He was not about to waste weeks or months getting to know someone to become friends with in order to finally have sex and realize they were incompatible for whatever reason. That was just plain dumb.

At a certain age, sex is no longer a mystery nor is it sacred. Basically, you like it or you don't. Into it or not. He reasoned that if sex was good, then friendship could follow. If not, it had been more fun finding out. Too many women had hang-ups of which he had no desire to be a part. George had it figured out. He pushed the send button.

Somewhere out in cyberspace his profile floated. Some would read it and be amused. Someone would send him a kiss. George felt confident. He had the online dating scene in his control. It was now only a question of time until he hooked the right one.

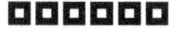

… TALL TALES TWO

Not All Days Are The Same

Regardless of who you are or where you came from, throughout the year, you are likely to have special days you remember, celebrate or would rather disappear from the calendar. The days and the reasons for their significance or aversion vary from person to person and from year to year. These are mine.

Halloween

I like Halloween. It is the best celebration of all, if that is the correct term. I have little interest in ghosts or goblins. I have forgotten the few witches that have crossed my path. I have no interest in the pagan rituals, which started the tradition. Halloween is much more than that to me.

It stems from when I was a child. Memories of that time, if they made you feel good, remain strong. Halloween starts as escapism in planning your costume so you can become someone or something else for at least one evening. In costume, only you know who you are. The rest are guessing at best. Days or weeks of preplanning add to the excitement. Get the costume right and you will have a good time.

Because I had no money to buy a costume, except maybe for a mask, my costume was created from what was available around the house. My grandmother would help me become a tramp with a painted face or a clown. A car accident victim wrapped with toilet paper and doused with ketchup was popular. An old bedsheet made one into a ghost. My preference was as a pirate. A patch over one eye, a bandana on my head, an old jacket three times too big for me, a bit of face paint and I was ready to terrorize the village.

I grew up in a small town with one main street lined with stores. On Halloween night, we could write on the windows with soap, forcing the owners to wash them the next day. A group of friends going from one store to the next, marking up the windows, was great fun at four and five years old. By six or seven, we had learned that soap was easily washed off. Dump the soap and use candles. Candle wax was far more difficult to remove. It actually took work. As you get older, you get smarter. At eight or nine years old, we went by the next day asking the owner if he wanted someone to clean the windows for a few bucks. We often got the job.

Tree-lined streets branched off the main street with residential homes on each side. Once we tired of marking windows, the real fun of Halloween, trick or treating, began. This entailed going door to door in our costumes saying 'trick or treat' to the residents who acted scared of our appearance and offered us treats. We held out our bags to be filled with assorted sweets.

How good it felt to be rewarded for our efforts. Returning home with the spoils of the night, we had enough candy to rot our teeth and make the dentist happy. Looking back, maybe he was the real winner of Halloween. In the morning, I would examine the goodies collected from the night before and wish that Halloween came more than once a year.

As I got older, Halloween remained the same but how one went about the celebration changed. In the high-school years, there was a Halloween dance in the gym with everyone in costume. Games were played, refreshments served, and of course dancing, with all events monitored by teachers. I had outgrown the pirate and instead, with the help of my aunt and her clothes, I became a girl for the night. No one knew who I was, with most thinking I was actually a female.

It had its advantages. Girls of that age tended to dance to rock and roll with other girls or in groups with boys. Dancing with another girl allowed the chance to brush against her in ways a boy could not. It was much more age satisfactory than writing on windows. An accidental grope here or a loose arm flying there, gathered useful information for a teenage boy.

Then there was Cabbage Night. It was popular in the northeast of the US on the night before Halloween, 30 October, during which young people played pranks and caused mischief in their neighborhoods. I was right into this with a few trusted friends. There was never a plan but after a few beers bought by a friendly drunk, a scheme developed.

Using one of their father's pick-up truck, the first stop was the local apple orchard where the picking season was in progress. A few cases of apples were 'appropriated' before taking a quick trip to the nearby town. With four or five of us in the back of the truck, the driver would roll through the center of town, or wherever the teens hung out, and we would pelt apples at anyone out in the open. It was over in minutes but provided many laughs.

Along the same lines, we would drive to known areas where those with cars took their girlfriends to 'park and make out.' If a car was found, we would bombard it with apples then disappear. On one occasion, it was the headmaster's son in his father's car. The car looked as if it had been in a hailstorm. The son was grounded. The villains were never caught.

Smoke bombs strategically placed were popular, as was ringing the minister's doorbell for him to find a burning paper bag on the porch. When he stomped on it, the fresh cow manure would cover his shoes. The good bit was that he could hear us laugh as we ran away. These activities made Halloween in a small town all the more anticipated.

Years later, I never lost my enthusiasm for this celebration. Whenever possible, I would organize a huge costume party knowing that people in costume lose their inhibitions and tend to get wilder than when in a business suit. Gone were the pranks of yesteryear. Instead, drugs and booze fueled behavior more intent on getting naked than disturbing someone.

That is not to say that someone usually said, "Why do I do that every year. I make the same mistake over and over. Shit! It felt good."

My daughter was two when she went on her first Halloween night of trick or treating. It was in LA as at that time we were living in Switzerland where Halloween is not celebrated. This tradition continued for many years and I remember that I enjoyed it as much as she did.

Later when she was in a private school in Australia, where Halloween is growing as an event, I had a party for all her class. The school heard about it and were concerned until they were assured there would be security with a dog. Adult supervision with no alcohol but costumes were mandatory.

Lighted pumpkins lined the driveway. Her thirty or so classmates arrived in various costumes to be welcomed by Frank N Furter himself, me. My daughter thought I was over the top. Many classmates were somewhat shocked at first but then settled into party mode. It was the talk of the school for weeks to come.

I guess after all these years, Halloween represents how I think and feel. It lets one be someone else for a period of time, to act differently with few restrictions. There are no expectations or demands. The very young, the old, and all in between can enjoy it. It can be whatever you want it to be and will give you pleasure. That can't be said of many things today.

Thanksgiving

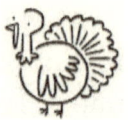

In my mind, there is a stark contrast between Thanksgiving and Christmas. Thanksgiving was always exciting to me. A day I looked forward to. There was no individual pressure. The test was to see how much you could eat. At our house, there was always plenty of food on the table for Thanksgiving. The traditional turkey, maybe a ham, all sorts of vegetables, and of course dessert. To cook the entire feast, my grandmother started the day before, making pies and cakes. Her was apple pie, my favorite, was accompanied by pumpkin pie and usually a lemon meringue pie. There would also be a chocolate cake and ice cream.

I liked to help my grandmother when she baked. I was very proficient at licking out the bowls, sticking my fingers into the frosting, and eating the apple slices before they reached the pie dish. She would scold me in a good-hearted way and let me continue. Knowing that I had played an integral part in the preparation of the dinner increased my enjoyment of Thanksgiving.

The meal itself was a casual affair with all relatives in the vicinity invited. I can never remember my mother or father being there but it is possible. There was lively conversation about the size of the turkey and the recent scandals in the small town where everyone knew everyone's business, or thought they did.

There was little talk of the meaning of Thanksgiving or of the Indians and Pilgrims. However, it was understood and appreciated that although we had very little money as a family, we had a feast as good or better than most hotels.

Living in Europe where they don't have Thanksgiving, because of my fond memories, I usually found a turkey, invited friends and celebrated whenever I was in the position to do so. I once sent a woman to buy a turkey and she returned with a six kilogram frozen turkey breast. I made the most of it, but for a person who prefers the legs and thighs, it was somewhat of a letdown. After that lesson learned, I went for the turkey myself. In Switzerland, in November, they are not easy to find.

Australia, the same as Europe, doesn't have Thanksgiving so I brought it with me. I concentrated on putting far more effort into that day in November than I ever did for Christmas. I guess it proves that the things you learned to like as a child you bring with you into adult life. The dislikes are more difficult to embrace and best avoided, forgotten and left behind.

On 16 November, I am walking through a mall decorated with fake trees, Christmas signs everywhere and an already tired looking Santa sitting and waiting to influence children to have their parents spend more than they can afford. I put the sights and sounds out of my head and think of stuffing the turkey that I am about to buy, if I can find the size I need.

It gives me pleasure to be inviting friends to a lunch or dinner with festive trimmings where all can eat, drink, and enjoy each other's company while I observe and am thankful for my memories of long ago.

Christmas

I have always disliked Christmas from the first time I can remember what it was all about. It has never varied throughout my life. I have often questioned why I have this aversion to this celebration without ever coming up with a clear answer. I am not sure if it is the Christmas season, the day itself, or how it makes me feel that is the underlying reason. I tend to think it is all of the above and more.

You may ask why a seven or eight-year-old child would dislike Christmas. For this age group it is the meant to be one of the most exciting days of the year. In order to try to comprehend why it was the opposite for me, we will go back to the time when I was that age.

My mother went in one direction and my father, the other, insuring there would be maximum distance between them. My brother and I were taken in by my grandmother, an unselfish, hardworking woman who was admired and respected by everyone in the small town where we grew up.

My father sent money from time to time for our support. My grandmother worked every day. I would describe the situation as lower middle class. There was always enough to eat and we never lacked for clothing. I rode my bike to school and ran wild with friends through fields and hills. I remember it as being a childhood of fun and adventure. That is until Christmas came around.

It was in the lead up, the first weeks of December that I started to feel uneasy. What would I get the family for gifts? I had saved pocket money and made money during the summer shagging golf balls. It was not about cost but that I never had any ideas of what to buy for anyone.

My grandmother and aunt, who lived in the house part-time, made a mammoth effort preparing for Christmas celebrations. A large fresh cut tree was decorated. A turkey ordered and all the trimmings added to make a feast. Everyone was buzzing with Christmas spirit except me. Whether I had done my shopping and the presents were wrapped and waiting to go under the tree or I was still struggling with what to buy for my brother, I felt sick. Not ready to vomit, although my stomach had an uneasy feeling, I was nervous and felt dread. Dread, meaning apprehension and fear. Why you ask? I don't know.

Santa came on Christmas Eve. On Christmas morning, most kids jumped from their beds, if they had managed to sleep, to stand before the tree in awe of what Santa had brought them. I wished I could stay in bed. At eight years old, the Santa charade was long past. My brother, four years younger, was still on the border of belief of who put the presents under the tree. At four, you tend to believe, fearing the presents might not appear if you didn't. I did my best to burst his bubble and make him cry. This was my revenge for Christmas making me feel so bad.

Everyone sat around the tree with my brother and I reading the names on the tags and passing out the presents. My grandmother always wrote 'from Santa' on the gifts she gave, which on reflection was a nice touch.

Later the adults in the family and any invited guests talked, generally discussing the gifts, before the women retired to the kitchen to prepare the turkey. I sat on the floor and looked over the presents I had opened. There were the normal things, underwear, socks, a shirt, pair of pants, maybe shoes. Then there were at least two toys that I had expressed interest in wanting. The best one usually from my aunt and the other from my grandmother. My attitude about the gifts was ho-hum. My relief that it was over was for another year, welcome.

That my parents were never present at Christmas didn't bother me in the least. I had basically forgotten about them, adopting myself in the sense that if I needed anything, I would be the one to get it. My grandmother was Catholic, so Christmas meant more church going. At nine-years old, I decided the church was a money-grabbing outfit that took change from kids and adults that they couldn't afford to part with. God had a nice house and many of them, all clean and warm. Why did he need my ten cents?

Allow me to add that I liked winter. I played in the snow and ice, skied and skated. It had nothing to do with the season that contributed to my dislike of 25 December.

The point at this juncture is that not family, upbringing, money, church, or God had any influence in making me dislike one of the favorite holidays of the year. As long as I lived at home, it never changed. It did not increase or lessen. It remained a constant over those years.

The years passed and examples of my Christmas behavior were evident. During my three years in the army, I stayed on base during all of the Christmas breaks. I never went on leave, volunteering to pull duty while others went home. I made excuses to avoid all Christmas parties. If I was with people I didn't know, I pretended Christmas was for them and therefore didn't affect me. Where others gathered to celebrate, I hid out preferring to be alone. There were times if a girlfriend invited me to a party during the holiday period and I couldn't weasel my way out of it, I put on a performance of conformity. On the outside, I was social while inside I was tied in knots counting the minutes until it was over.

On rare occasions where I knew what present someone would like, giving it to them eased the anxiety to some extent. Most of the time, I never knew what to get, leaving it to the last hour, and then in panic bought something they didn't want or need. This made the whole process worse. The dread would last until New Year.

Sometime in my mid-twenties, my dislike of New Year's Eve became the same as my feeling for Christmas. I really cannot remember ever having a great New Year's Eve. Maybe I did, but don't remember. I do recall being at parties where everyone was pretending to have a good time. Then in unison at the stroke of midnight, they blew paper whistles in your ear and kissed you. I tried to dodge the kisses and still appear happy even though I was really bored.

A good time to me was being in bed with someone likeminded, sipping champagne or pouring it over each other before midnight, enjoying a long night together. It took me a few years to realize that I didn't need New Year's Eve to have fun. I could get crazy any day I chose.

It occurred to me that Christmas and New Year's Eve were now the festive season in my mind. Instead of disappearing for a couple of days, it meant a couple of weeks. On 20 December, my dream was for the 10 January.

In my early thirties, I started a ski business at a winter resort in Switzerland. The winter season is from when it snows maybe mid-November until Easter, whenever that arrives. A season of less than twenty weeks to make a living to survive fifty-two. The most important time of the year is, you guessed it, Christmas. The crowd arrives after 20 December and stays until 10 January. Twenty days or so that can make or break your season.

How does this relate to my dislike for this period of the year? In a service business like we had, you have to be friendly, and in our case, very friendly. This entailed skiing with the clients and partying with them. In return, they spent up in the shop and brought their friends. You were obliged to say, 'Merry Christmas' and then 'Happy New Year'.

That doesn't seem like it involves any effort, in fact it is quite normal. Not for me. At first, I said it, without thinking, to people or clients I knew and liked. To others I tried to avoid saying it. As the years went on, I could not say it. It became a game for me to meet or serve clients during the festive period and find a way to be friendly without mentioning those words. I would say, 'enjoy the parties', 'happy holidays', 'all the best to you'. Anything but Merry Christmas. Saying it made me feel like I had been slapped in the face with a silk handkerchief. It was not meant to hurt, it was just a reminder you had done something wrong. Finding a way to not say it to a close friend while making them feel you were interested was part of the challenge. Today I doubt if anyone ever suspected.

Moving on to the time I was married, my wife knew of my thoughts and thought I was crazy. I tried to temper my distaste when in a group or party, by suffering in silence. She was well aware of the word game as she worked with me in a new chocolate and fine-wine business. I often told her it's only two weeks. The rest of the year, I'm perfect. You are way ahead.

Then our daughter was born. Now I could see a dilemma looming. I didn't want to spoil her Santa and Christmas enjoyment because of my mindsets. When she was twenty-months old, a friend who dressed as Santa offered to drop by our place on Christmas Eve. We had the house decorated and a small tree with lights. The spirit of the holidays. My daughter was sitting peacefully on the floor when Santa arrived. One look at the man and she started screaming. My wife thought that he had scared her. She continued to cry until Santa left. I smiled. My daughter took after me.

From that time on until she was over the hoax at about six-years old, I played the Christmas game. It was the only time I truly made an effort. It was easier than I expected to adjust to being the family man with spirit and dance around the tree only because I knew it was an act. It also made it easy because I was sure in my daughter's mind she didn't care at all about Christmas. I knew that because whatever gifts she received, she was bored in a day or so. The large box that the refrigerator came in, she played with for months. She knew it had nothing to do with Christmas.

Today she agrees with me that the whole Christmas thing is best ignored. We do not exchange presents. We enjoy a good meal like any other day and give presents when we want, not when we are obligated.

Over the years, I have been in relationships during the festive twenty-day period. How did the person I was involved with handle my indifference to the holidays? Not always with understanding. I warned them of my feelings months in advance. Like so many things, they hear what they want and then are surprised when you say you don't want a present, are not giving any and refuse to go out on New Year's Eve.

I am not one for tension at any time when it can be avoided. The best way to escape this sort of stress is pre-planning. Send the better half to visit their family. Go on a vacation so the present is the vacation and you are where you know no one. When nothing else comes to mind, acquire the dreaded winter flu at just the right time and watch games on television in peace while the in-laws in another house throw turkey bones at each other.

In the twilight of my dislike of Christmas, I think that I am unusual in that while most people look forward to holidays with time off work, getting together with family and friends, and maxing out the credit cards buying gifts, I suffer through weeks of torment. Day after day, I am racked with guilt and anxiety for which there is no cure. In silence, for the most part, I endure where I am convinced most would falter. Of course, on the bright side of this comes February and I DO NOT receive several credit card bills with amounts over $3,000 that can be paid off in minimal payments over thirty years at 22.8%! Total repayment of only $11,671 or something like that on each card.

The secret to one's well-being over a long period is to be happy with yourself and live alone.

Alternatively, find someone who understands you and accepts you for what you are. Not liking Christmas can be a deal breaker in many circumstances. Some would label such a person as being unpatriotic or sacrilegious. I am pleased to announce that I have found someone who is far more sympathetic. My simple dislike for Christmas is trivial compared to my other slip-ups, flaws, shortcomings, lapses, imperfections and burdens she puts up with on a daily basis.

It is said that with age you mellow or get over things. Perhaps I have, but 25 December can still be a time of fear and loathing in my mind. With the help of someone who cares, the dread has subsided to some degree, and it's just another day for me. No anticipations, no expectations.

Maybe in reading this you will have figured out what or why I have spent my life disliking Christmas. I must admit I remain as baffled as I ever was.

Birthdays

The unique thing about birthdays is that everybody has one. After that, it becomes ho-hum for the most part. I am sure many make a special commitment to celebrate their birthday. From blowing out the first candle, to sipping champagne, to trying to blow out more candles than you have wind for, to being wheeled up to a table containing a cake with your name on it, the birthday ritual goes on throughout life.

Personally, I liked it slightly more than I disliked Christmas. There were two advantages. One was that I didn't have to think and buy anything for anyone. Secondly, I was alone on the receiving end.

My day but not always my way. On my sixth birthday, my parents arranged a party for me and invited all my first-grade class. It was held at my father's hotel. A friend had a fair ride set up in the massive dining room for all the kids to enjoy. Games were played including a peanut hunt. My mother wouldn't let me participate for a reason that was not made clear to my six-year old mind. Of course, I threw a fit. It ruined my party. From that point on, my birthday held an unpleasant memory.

In the following years, I tried to hide from the day but those around me always reminded me. I smiled and said thank you for any gifts. I hid the contempt I felt. When I was older and on my own, I forgot about my birthday. I never told anyone, therefore never had well-wishers or presents. I also convinced myself that if I didn't acknowledge my birthday, I didn't get any older.

I didn't let how I regarded my birthday carryover to others. I was quick to buy presents and help friends celebrate their birthdays. If they enjoyed it, who was I to dampen the fest.

Birthdays come and go. A curious phenomenon happens as the numbers go up. The number becomes more important than the day. For example at age sixteen, you almost become an adult meaning you can now put into practice what you have been thinking of since age thirteen, without going to jail.

At age eighteen, you can drink legally in some places, vote and join the army without your parent's consent. Age twenty-one. Now, that is the BIG one. More of everything to celebrate. Bigger party, more booze, exciting sex, and hopes that you can remember what really happened. To top it off you now have all adult rights and responsibilities.

The next years go back to being ordinary birthdays until the number ends with a zero. The dreaded zero. It means you're getting old. You getting old? How does that happen? You are bulletproof or thought you were. Is that a wrinkle by your eye? No, not a receding hairline. My breasts are the same as when I was eighteen, or are they? Only one piece of cake, I will drink less, expect more expensive presents, and be sure to have sex. I read somewhere if you don't have sex on your birthday you will have a year of bad luck in love. True or not, there is no reason to risk it.

Forty, the big four zero. That is a number in the parade of birthdays that strikes fear. Fear varies depending who has reached that point. For some it is the realization at a friend's funeral that if they can die, so can I. Many ponder the number and relate that to it being the halfway point of their life. My life is half over. What happened to the years?

Some think about what they have accomplished. Two divorces, alimony to pay, out of a job, never found love, still living at home, a loving family but on the verge of bankruptcy, or being super rich but lonely and depressed. The most popular is the well-rehearsed lament, I have achieved so many goals but there is so much more to do and so little time. Life is unfair. If it takes anyone forty years to realize that life is unfair, there is little hope for them.

Now comes the nine years of only admitting your age to those who know. Birthday parties are smaller affairs. The number is seldom mentioned except when you receive a card in the mail with a huge forty-seven on the front and a remark inside saying, 'If wrinkles are experience lines, you should be at the head of the class. Happy Birthday.' You should never have considered that person a friend!

The next zero that comes into your life is the one that passes with little fanfare. Fifty is not old and not young. It is just confusing. It feels like sixty in the morning but forty when playing sport and thirty-five when someone attractive catches your eye.

When once the attractive one would flash you a smile, they now look straight through you as if you're not there. You are a ghost to them. Self-esteem tumbles as confusion intensifies. You rush to the magnifying mirror to examine yourself. Your reflection looks great. You strut from the bathroom feeling your confidence returning. Now where are my glasses so I can check Facebook!

Sixty is the zero that demands decisions. Decisions of all sizes and complexities. Some never previously been considered and others that have been put off for too long. There is no putting them in order of importance and dealing with them in an organized way. They are not like in times gone by when the questions were simple. Which university should I go to? Is that the car for me? Should I marry her or admit that I maybe gay? The mood you were in on any given day defined which assessment you would tackle.

At sixty, it's about wills, cosmetic surgery, hair dye, retirement planning, funeral arrangements, medical cover, and who will love me when I'm sixty-four.

Not All Days Are The Same

Seventy is the new fifty, I heard someone say. I think they were trying to cheer up Grandma. Seventy means you can take some pleasure in that you have outlived someone in your school class. Unfortunately, you know that person who picked on you and stole your girl or boyfriend lives on and you have to outlive that bastard. Some retire and soon die of boredom. Others enjoy life in retirement homes. Still a few pass the days in Asia or the Philippines with a nimble young one accommodating all the pleasures Viagra promises. So many choices at seventy and soooo little time.

Eighty, and here only the ones with full or close to full functions of the body and mind will be counted. Once out of bed, the thought of the day is guessing how many more times you will do this. How will I die? Where? Who will care?

Ah! Toast soaked in white coffee and seventeen vitamins swallowed one after another with a glass of water. What a chore. Now where was I? Oh, yes. Have I paid the funeral insurance? Shit, they cancelled it because they say I'm too old. Is that the phone or is it the microwave telling me where I left last night's dinner. I need a nap.

Ninety. I'm ready. You don't scare me. Bring it on!

Valentine's Day

What's not to like? Why not celebrate. Everyone loves a box of chocolates and a dinner date. You can forget a birthday or anniversary but the stores and the television advertisements remind you of Valentine's Day so you never forget. Whatever your age, it is a good excuse to get laid. What person can refuse after you have remembered them with a gift, paid for a night out, and you are on your best behavior.

There is no doubt that Valentine's Day rates above Teachers' Day, Bring Your Child To Work Day, Forest Fire Prevention Day, or Columbus's birthday. There should be two Valentine's Days each year. I propose to put that on the ballot.

The first day of fishing

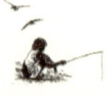

The first day of fishing, 1 May in Vermont, was my favorite day of the year from the age of six to sixteen. I planned this occasion like a military operation. My pole with reel was ready to go. I had enough hooks and sinkers. Days beforehand, I dug up earthworms and kept them in a box of soil until the day arrived. I checked and rechecked all of my equipment many times.

Then I started thinking about where I would go to start fishing. I knew all the best spots. I had to decide which one was the right place to cast my line at daybreak. How many others might be there? Would the fish be bigger in spot X or spot Z? To answer these important questions, inspection of the sites was required more than once in the days before the season opened.

The clear water in the streams allowed me to see the trout easily. At each place, as I watched them swim against the current from the bank or a bridge, I counted the number as best I could and estimated their size. I knew my final decision as to where to go would only be made on the morning. Weather would play an important part so I had to watch the weather report and be prepared to change if the report was revised.

The best time to fish for trout was early morning, early evening just before dusk or during a thunderstorm when food was washed into the streams by heavy rain. The middle of the day was a waste of time. Trout were smart but I considered myself smarter.

It was difficult going to sleep in the nights leading up to the big day. On the night before, it was almost impossible as I worried I would oversleep and not be out the door at daybreak, which was around five o'clock. This was pure excitement. I knew I was a good trout fisherman. I had been taught by the best, my grandfather, who had also handmade my rod. It was an Orvis rod. One of the best at that time and even more famous today. He worked for Orvis for many years.

If the first day of fishing fell on a school day I would be absent from class. If my teacher or principal called, my grandmother always made an excuse for me. As the pattern became apparent it was assumed I would be a no-show on the first day of fishing. I was not alone. Four or five of my fishing friends followed my example with or without their parent's knowledge.

The limit you were allowed to catch in one day was twelve trout, each having to be at least six inches long. I set a target of six trout at least ten inches long. Under that length, I usually threw them back. Great fishermen do not keep small fish. To the best of my memory there were very few times when I did not achieve my target and usually returned home with a basket of ten or so brown or native trout, many longer than twelve inches.

My grandmother would fry up the catch and all of us would enjoy the meal. I would brag to my grandfather and he would say he taught me well. Christmas might be for Santa but the first day of fishing was mine.

Not All Days Are The Same

Other days during the year that may be anticipated without having the same effect as those already mentioned are the day the fair came to town; the day the swimming pool opened; the first big snow storm of the year or the next time you drank when you were sixteen regardless of how sick it made you feel.

For each individual, not all days are the same.

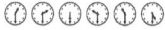

TALL TALES TWO

Off the Grid

Thomas Whelan is my friend and has been for over forty years. We have traveled together, shared houses, smoked plenty of dope, been to athletic events, and most importantly, had great times in each other's company.

Tom now lives in California. Many, many years ago, he bought a home overlooking the ocean. That the cost was more than he could afford at the time didn't stop him from buying exactly what he wanted. I am sincerely glad he made that decision, as in the ensuing years I have called his place my second home, staying there while visiting Tom, at least two or three times a year. It has felt like home besides being a stopover for the many trips that began there and weeks later ended up there.

Soon after the house was purchased, Tom called in an architect friend to completely update the interior. The changes on the inside were outstanding and the hot tub located on a deck off the main bedroom took advantage of the breathtaking views of the shoreline. A concealed wine cellar and small bar provided the refreshments needed to accompany the bubbles in the hot tub.

To go to Gelsons, perhaps one of the world's most expensive grocery stores, to replenish supplies, Tom had a variety of flash machines. A Corvette, Porsche, and other convertibles shared the space in his garage. Life was good for Tom. It was my pleasure to share the lifestyle whenever I visited, letting me have the run of the house. Tom lent me his Porsche and put up with waking up to strange ladies rushing to the toilet or standing nude looking out over the ocean with a coffee in one hand and joint in the other.

Tom and his brother Paul were the third generation born to the successful Whelan family. The grandparents had started with a small store in a strip mall. Soon they owned the mall and moved seriously into real estate, particularly building and renting mall space. Their parents took over the business when the grandparents died and it eventually passed on to Tom and his brother.

This is a good time to look at some facts. Around seven in ten families lose their fortune by the second generation. By the third generation, the figure has jumped to almost ninety percent. The most compelling causes as to why or how this happens is that younger family members are ill prepared or unwilling to shoulder the responsibility and hard work that it takes to maintain their prosperity. In spite of expensive educations, they grow up in surroundings with plenty of money without the work ethic required to continue the success.

Sometimes the fortunes are diluted among too many family members or the family member who takes over the business has no real interest and turns it over to long-time family lawyers, accountants, and well-paid advisers. They are non-trusting of outsiders and have the feeling people are after their money or out to exploit them.

The fear that friends only like them for their money also plays on their mind, increasing their paranoia. To top it off, there is always pressure to be better or more successful than the parents before them.

There are other instances where the fortune was blown through family squabbles and divorces, or on frivolous items such as cars, planes, and parties. The Vanderbilts, Pulitzers, and Hartfords are but a few that saw fortunes disappear over the generations for many of the above reasons.

To a lesser extent, the Whelans were not in this category but are an example of the behavior. Neither of the brothers had any interest in taking over the day-to-day running of the business, instead leaving it in the hands of trusted family officials while they escaped the climate of the mid-west and headed to California and the allure of La La Land.

Paul and Tom both graduated from universities in California. Paul got married and had a large family while dabbling in investments using the substantial income derived from the business. No venture were long term nor did they increase his wealth. They kept him busy with a title that changed when the next scheme developed. Paul returned monthly to the offices of the family business for a sit down with the advisors to insure they kept the cash flowing in his direction.

Tom worked for a few years before deciding travel was his main interest. Europe, Hawaii, cruises to all corners of the globe, and trips with friends who had the time to accompany him. When his friends settled down and became involved with work and family, Tom went to visit them.

One of his close friends lived in Europe. He would spend two winter months with her and her family at their home in a ski resort. I lived in this resort and the same family were friends of mine. This is how I first met Tom. Our friendship grew and over the years, and whenever possible, I was the one who accompanied him on trips.

Tom fell in love and was married. It was doomed from the start for a variety of better-forgotten reasons and a divorce quickly followed. Everyone agreed he was lucky in avoiding a massive Californian settlement in an agreement that sent her packing and Tom free.

Regarding the business, Tom was much less interested than Paul. Because having a family gave Paul a much greater need for income than Tom, he proposed a buy-out to pay Tom an agreed amount, every month for life. Tom signed the deal.

Because the house sat on a cliff that was slowing sliding away whenever the fall rains came, Tom had to spend serious money shoring it up. Pillars driven deep into the ground would save the house. Half of the front yard had already slipped away causing the hot tub and much of the deck to be removed. A new smaller deck was constructed. He gave the house a makeover, to freshen up the interior décor. With renovations completed, Tom was back on the road of travel and vacations.

Paul left his wife and kids in a nasty divorce. He had found a new love and between them, their 'new' family had almost as many kids as the Brady Bunch. Paul did not fare as well as Tom had in his divorce. He was up for an alimony payment of six figures, every year, for the rest of his ex-wife's life.

Years passed and nothing much changed in the lives of the Whelan boys. One a self-styled entrepreneur generating no additional income while suffering one bad investment after another. The other continued on his merry way. Two months in Europe, two months in Hawaii in the spring and another two in the fall. There was no reason to be in LA in less than perfect weather.

As I mentioned, I spent a few weeks a year staying at the house. It was a reason to go to LA as well as a stopping off point on my way back and forth to Hawaii from Europe. It was because of Tom knowing Maui so well that made me interested in Hawaii. I was into windsurfing. Maui was the mecca.

The first year I was there, Tom and I shared a house with a couple of other friends from Europe. Life was good for all concerned. After that, I went back to Maui every summer for the next ten years. Tom was there for most of that time.

I ended up permanently moving from Europe to Hawaii where I lived for five years before moving on to Australia. Tom visited me in Australia, toured the country and spent time in New Zealand. I made many trips to LA, staying with him while my daughter was in school in California. Being able to stay with Tom saved me thousands of dollars, saying nothing of the fun we had. Movies, restaurants, and a shared political outlook made us close.

A couple of years ago, Tom told me the family business was not going very well. Shops were closing, leaving too much space unrented. The downturn in the economy was the cause with high hopes things would improve as the crisis ended. Tom told me Paul was worried. I suggested that maybe he should sell it all. The answer was that it was the wrong time. He would not get the right price. That was where the conversation ended.

Six months ago, the shit hit the fan. I was staying with Tom when he told me that his brother could no longer pay him the agreed monthly amount. He could only pay a third. This would soon leave Tom broke as he had very high mortgage repayments. I was surprised to hear that after all the years of having the house, it was still mortgaged and found out it was due to borrowing to keep the house from falling down the cliff. It was likely that Tom was heading towards defaulting on the loan.

As I saw it, there were three courses of action.

1. Sue his brother and make him sell his house. This Tom would not do.
2. Have Paul sell the family business, which would be a fire sale. Or,

3. Tom would have to sell his home after forty years.

We arranged a meeting with three of Tom's closest friends who all had his interests at heart. Tom immediately ruled out option one and two. Selling his house was the only way out that he could see.

I have worked in real estate for fifteen years being a high-volume seller and a developer. I outlined a plan that I felt was his best chance to sell at the price he needed. There were many things to consider.

The house was very much in need of repairs as nothing had been done on the interior or exterior in years. It sat on a cliff with a direct drop of 300 feet to the road below. That would eliminate families with small children. That the house had been pillared to stop the sliding would scare off older people once they read the report. The scope of who might buy it was narrow. The main draw cards were the one-of-a-kind views to the ocean and the coastline to the south.

Other houses nearby had sold for over three million. Tom wanted $3.5 million. He had the bank to pay off, thirty-eight percent Californian sales tax on capital gains, and the commission. The amount left would be the sum he had to live on for the rest of his life. With a $3.5 million sale, the net Tom could receive might be about $800 thousand.

My idea was to give it to Sotheby's or another high international profile realtor with hopes of selling unseen to an offshore cashed-up buyer. The others agreed this was a good plan. The buyers would trust Sotheby and be dazzled by the view in the photos or video.

Tom told his brother who informed him he should use his son as the agent. Tom said his brother would be pissed off if he didn't use the son. I told him his nephew was no doubt a good guy, however, selling his house at the price he wanted, with the obvious problems, took someone with powerful international standing.

A one-man operation would not get the required results. Tom dismissed our suggestions and signed on with his nephew. I felt no good would come from this decision. I was convinced, without pure luck, there was no way in hell the house would sell for close to that price.

Over the next four months, there were a number of offers in the three million dollar range. They all backed out once they read the soil report. Tom was in panic mode. Finally, he insisted that his nephew engage a realtor with more experience. Within two weeks, there were two more offers but they were for less than three million. One offer cancelled. The other was a builder who knew the problems of the area and had the ability to do whatever was needed building wise. He offered $2.4 million.

I was in contact with Tom by phone from Australia when he told me of the offer and that it would very likely go unconditional. I decided to go to LA to talk with Tom about what he had in mind once it sold and spend my last time at the house.

Tom had decided, when the house sold, he wanted to rent in the same area he now lived. The problem was that at $2.4 million, after everything was paid, he would clear less than $500,000. With rents around $5,000 a month, it was clear he could not afford it. He would have to move to a less expensive area, preferably out of California, away from its high prices and taxes.

I suggested he think about moving to Nevada or New Mexico. When that was rejected, I suggested farther south where the prices were half the cost of the area he wanted to move to. Again, Tom was determined to stay in close proximity to where he had been for so long.

When someone has lived in the same house for over forty years, they have collected many things with emotional attachments and memories. There are also many books, clothes, garage junk, and clutter that goes unnoticed until it's time to pack it up and move it out.

Tom had no children. He told me that leaving the house was like losing a child. It was a sentiment that I could understand. What was more important to me was that unless he changed his lifestyle or died, he was looking at being broke in about five years. This bothered me as I could envision him pushing a shopping cart with a couple of bags hanging off it near the Santa Monica pier. Not a pretty sight.

I tried again. "You have to get out of LA and better yet, out of California. Go to Nevada or New Mexico where it is cheap."

"I want to stay here. My friends are here. I know my way around."

"You have no friends here. Your friends are all over the place and you communicate by phone. Nothing would change."

"No, I will find something here."

"Think about this. On the $2.4 million sale, you are paying just over one million in tax. One million dollars. Don't pay the tax. I wouldn't. You would have to pay it in about eight months when you do your taxes but by then you could have disappeared. The chance of getting caught are slim and none. In the event you did, you'd pay a fine or better yet, you'd say you blew the money. What will they do, put you in jail? If so, good. Free dental, medicine, TV, and you can order in food. All in a gated community!"

"I could never do that. I am too afraid."

"As I see it, you have little choice. I've sold homes in a few places and left without paying any tax. I'm not in jail."

"Yeah, that was years ago. Things are different now. Everything is computerized. They will get you."

"No. Not a chance if you make a plan. You move out of state, change your name, get a new driving license, dump the credit cards and pay cash. Thomas Whelan disappears. You tell your friends you are on vacation which is normal for you and you contact them by phone, cell phone only."

"You're serious?"

"Of course. I'll help you. A million bucks is a million bucks. Better you have it than this fucked up state giving it to illegals."

"I'm too old for that sort of thing."

"A million bucks in cash in your pocket. Think about that."

"I will ask my accountant."

"Are you crazy? He's been taking your money for years. The well is running dry for him. Never speak to him."

"I can pretend I am asking for a friend."

"As if he would believe that. Forget him. He has taken you for enough. I have a plan that puts a million in your pocket. All you have to do is agree, keep your mouth shut and follow the plan."

"I can't. I would get caught."

"Maybe, but you are also too young not to do it. Pushing a shopping cart with a Gelson's bag is not all that unlikely in a few years."

I let the conversation go. I had planted the idea. It was all I could do.

Two weeks later Tom received a letter with the provisional payout shown to include all taxes, deductions, fees, commissions, and payout owed the bank. The figure was a dismal $447,612. For a person who could expect to live at least another ten years that was about $44,000 a year. The apartment Tom had found and intended to rent was $48,000 a year without services, which he could probably manage if he didn't eat, drive a car or use electricity.

As he stood there in shock, I pushed a number in front of him.

$943,600.

"In your hand if you DO NOT pay the tax. Think about it!"

Tom sat still looking at the paper. "I'm fucked."

"You are if you allow it. At some point in the life, the moment arrives when you have to step up and out of your comfort zone. This is that time for you. You play by the book and for sure, you will end up in a place unknown and uncomfortable for you. Take charge, play a new game and fuck them."

"You think I should do that?"

"There is no thought involved. You have little choice. I'm here to help you. It's a new adventure like we did in the old days except now we play more serious."

"How do you know what to do?"

"I've been doing it all my life. I never play by rules if I can avoid it. How do you think I bought all those homes? Completely manufactured the documents that the banks wanted to see. Today it is just as easy. Give me the word and you will be almost half a million richer."

"I don't know. I am too old. I could go to jail. It is different today. They get you with the computers. You are wrong. They would jail me."

"You could die and not have to worry about it. That is one choice. Go out and jump off the cliff. Fly until you hit the road and a semi-trailer squashes you. Another possibility is for you tell me what is important to make you happy for the rest of your days. It cannot be a place in LA or even California and I will make it happen. I will need your help but together we will have you continue the good life with certain restrictions."

"What restrictions?"

"First, you do not say a word to your brother of your plans. NOTHING. That also goes for the friends you chat with on the phone. You're selling and taking a vacation before deciding where to live. That's it. No other information. It may be hard to be out of contact but that is a small price to pay at first. Is this clear?"

"I understand that."

"Good. You mention anything to anyone except that you are going on vacation and there is no plan. No contact! You will not be able to travel out of the US. You will not have a passport, as you will no longer be Thomas Whelan. Travel where you like including Hawaii but stay in the US."

"I will be someone else?" Tom thought about that. "I never imagined being someone else."

"You will have a new identity, a new name, new ID. That's all. It will mean a low profile. No credit cards, no banks, a cash life, which is better in any case. You rent, have a family-type car and use cell phones to call your friends. You say you're traveling, in Hawaii or wherever. Very little changes from now except you are not in this house or in LA."

"What is my new name?"

"Whatever you want. You could go with Frank Abagnale, the guy from the film 'Catch Me If You Can'. That would be funny. How about Frank Fortune? That has a nice ring."

"You're joking?"

"Not at all my friend. You tell me you are into this and I will make it happen. The best part is that I won't charge you a cent for my expertise."

"Real nice of you. Will you visit me in jail?"

"Hell no. I don't hang out with jail birds or crims who defraud the government."

"I expected that."

I had intended to return home but changed my mind and stayed with Tom. Two weeks before the settlement and after much discussion, Tom told me that I was right, "Half a million is a lot of money to give to the state to waste. Reluctantly I'll go with your plan. What exactly is that plan?"

Tom was a man who had spent most of his life without a moment of stress. I could see on his face that this had changed. The moving was a major undertaking both physically and mentally. Now with agreeing to cut the state out of the tax had him close to breaking.

I walked towards him holding a glass of champagne, "Here my friend. One of your best bottles to celebrate a new life. I know this has you stressed out. I understand it's hard to avoid. You have to think of this in a different light. Remember the time when you thought you would lose a bundle in the divorce and how uptight you were. Or when you were skiing in that shit snow, and swore so much we thought you would have a heart attack. All of that passed and you survived. This is no different, just dealing with another adventure. Two months from now you will open another bottle and raise a toast to your good decision."

"You sure?"

"I don't get involved with things that are not a success. This is an adventure. One that is better than most as we are fucking the great state of California out of money they would just blow on some liberal cause. You are the best cause I know of to blow the money on. Agree?"

"Cheers."

I sat down beside Tom and explained the plan.

The first part was to create a new identity. I knew a man from skiing days who knew another who for $200 could come up with a social security card in the name of Frank Fortune. Frank Fortune now had a utility bill made out to him from a rental apartment in Marina Del Rey. A photocopier, an internet letterhead and there was the bill. Two forms of identity were enough to score an international driver's license so Frank could drive. That was the first part of my involvement. Within three days, we had the identity.

Now it was Tom's turn. He would pay off and close all of his credit cards, as well as cancel his insurance policies. We drove together and sold his car for cash. He then rented a car in the name of Frank Fortune. Tom closed out one of his bank accounts. The other he kept open to receive the settlement from the house. An estate sale was planned to sell the furnishings that were no longer needed. Things that were dear to Tom were set aside to be shipped somewhere.

Where to live was an endless discussion. This was perhaps the most difficult decision for Tom. Agreeing to become Frank Fortune was far less awkward than finding a destination to live. I suggested Vegas as it had a large temporary population making it easier to become 'lost'. A small city like Santa Fe was nice but too small. A large place like Phoenix, Arizona was too hot. Back and forth it went.

"Look Frank, wherever you go you don't have to stay there forever. If you don't like it, move."

"I want to be settled. I don't want to feel that I'm on the run. I want a nice place that I like."

Time was running out. There was much to be done. Finally, I decided to take charge.

"Frank, enough of this bullshit about where to live. You can choose jail or a place where you will fit in with a million others and no one will notice. The place for you is Miami, Florida. Surprisingly it has the largest transient population in America. It's cheap, nice weather, beaches, great Cuban cigars, and an abundance of rentals. A two-bedroom beachfront furnished or unfurnished from $1,800 a month is far better than $4,200 in LA nowhere near the beach. I'll fly to Miami and find something. Once the house settles, we can then rent a U-Haul truck and drive there with all of your gear. Think about it. You will be lost in the white-shoe crowd."

"That worries me. Miami. I never thought about it. I will look online. Miami. That could be a good idea."

"You have till morning when I'll book a flight and go find you a place to live."

I flew to Miami and looked at a dozen apartments before settling on a three-bedroom fourth-floor oceanfront unit in a secure complex. It was unfurnished with a huge balcony, and two full bathrooms. The complex had two pools and a gym. There was a mall within walking distance. I paid a deposit and flew back to LA.

"It has all you want, gym and pools plus three bedrooms. Great view and close to shopping. There is an antenna on the roof for a choice of cable companies. I like the price. $2,200 a month. Look at the photos."

"Looks good. Will I like it?"

"You've already taken it. I paid the deposit. You will love it."

"But will I like Miami? That worries me. I guess I can get used to it."

"You stay there a while and then if you don't like it, you move. Go to Texas. Wherever you like."

Paul was interested in what Tom had in mind as to where he was going to live. They talked on the phone. I had instructed Tom to say little about his plans except to mention that he may take a vacation to Europe to cope with the stress of the sale. My real worry was that after the sale when Paul knew Tom had the cash, he would come and ask for a loan. Tom being Tom would give him the money. It was important to get Tom on vacation as quickly as possible after the sale.

The estate sale had been huge. Because I had taken the measurements of the Miami apartment, he kept the things that would fit and sold the surplus furnishings. Surprisingly most of the items sold at good prices. The cash at the end of the day surprised Tom. What remained unsold, he gave away.

Settlement day duly arrived. Tom went to the realtor's offices to sign the paperwork. I returned the rental car and rented a medium sized U-Haul truck. I also engaged two of the gardeners who previously looked after Tom's yard, to load the truck. They worked most of the day carefully moving the furniture into the truck and stowing it for the drive.

Tom went from the settlement to his bank informing them that a large sum of money would be transferred to his account. He also advised his banker he was going to move to Seattle to be closer to his son. He would return to the bank in two days and wanted the entire amount in cash. The banker said his piece about the dangers of carrying so much cash and how the bank would be happy to look after it for him.

Tom said, "Thank you but please have it ready when I return."

Tom was worried about how to deal in cash only. I explained that he would buy a safe and have it installed in the apartment. He would take the amount of cash he needed each day and the rest would be safe in the safe. PayPal could be used to pay some bills, others in cash. He would use burn phones with prepaid cards and pay the condominium directly for his electricity. Going all cash was easier than he thought.

We sat in the backyard and drank champagne as we spoke of the memories that were in the walls of the house. We watched the sun set into the ocean. It was sad as well as exciting. Try as one might, nothing lasts forever, even a house that has meant so much. The new owner was going to demolish and rebuild it on a safe secure foundation. On the bright side, it would have a new lease of life and bring happiness to more generations.

We drank to the thought of life going on; of Thomas disappearing; of Frank Fortune stepping into the picture, knowing he has the means to live as he is accustomed; of fucking over the state of California before they could get to him.

I parked down the road from the bank and waited. I could see Frank approaching with a Gelson's shopping bag in each hand.

"All counted and in the bags," said Frank as he put the bags behind the seat of the truck and climbed into the cab. He then turned to me and said, "Hit the road Jack."

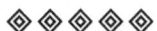

BEING AN AUTHOR

Let me start by saying I never intended to become an author. As I remember, I had no plan to be anything. In that endeavor, I would say I have been an overwhelming success.

Life as it turned out, handed me skills that came in good use more by accident than choice. I was a good talker. That allowed me to be a good salesman. I also had the ability to understand that when a product did not sell, I could find a way to manipulate the product or the circumstance to make it sellable. Successful businesses were the result of this.

The first thought of anything to do with writing, except on an occasional postcard, was when I was living with a wealthy woman in Europe. I had no job or income that was evident. To avoid embarrassment when the question, 'what do you do?' came up, I gave myself employment as a freelance magazine journalist. I would explain to whoever was rude enough to ask the question in the first place, that although it sounded exciting, the job was really boring, covering stories that for the most part were mundane. The conversation ended at that point.

One day for some unknown reason, I decided that since I was a journalist, I should write a story. There was a typewriter in the house. I bought some paper and proceeded to write a story called Lopez, about a baseball pitcher. The year was around 1965 or 1966. The story had 5,961 words. I know this because I carried the sheets of paper around with me until 2016. I have no photos at all from this time of my life, only this story. It must have been some kind of fate since I reworked this tale and added it as one of the short stories in my first book of short stories, TALL TALES.

That was the only time I had any inclination for writing more than a postcard or a letter to my grandmother and aunt. This only happened a few times a year and went as follows:

Hello,

Hope all is well with you. I am well and having fun. There is, (depending on the season) plenty of snow or it has been good weather here.

I am skiing a lot, traveling a lot, or changed my car, moved house, no longer with Gina (as the situation called for).

I will write soon. Hello to all.

Jack

This was the extent of my writing until my Grandmother died. After that, my output was down by half.

In 1992, I left Europe after thirty years, moving first to Maui for five years and then to Australia where I have been since 1995. I divorced, raised a daughter as a single parent and sold real estate before going into the development of high-end waterfront homes.

During my whole life, I was able to spot opportunities, act on them, be successful until I was bored and then move onto something else. This is an exciting way of doing things but has its drawbacks. People acquire wealth from being in one place doing the same thing over a long period of time. Values goes up, they cash out and go off into the sunset drinking margaritas. I would leave a business selling it for less than its future value then not work until the next opportunity came along. In the meantime I'd party the money away and be back to start again.

I watched my former business partners become rich while I had all fun. What is the price one can put on fun and adventures? Ask ten people, you will get ten answers. I would not trade my life with anyone. In my mind, I was living every day while others merely existed.

I have played cards since I was four. My father ran games in his hotel. He played with me sometimes. I played my way through the army making more money at cards than the army salary. In St. Moritz, I played gin rummy, bridge, and backgammon. While that might sound like I was a gambler, I was not. I was good and usually won by knowing my limits. When Texas Holdem gained world attention as the game of the moment, I started playing in Australia.

I met Neil, a computer wizard, who was starting a poker company simply because he could. He was not a front man or a salesman. I saw a chance and we became partners in Gold Coast Poker. We ran free poker in clubs and pubs where we were paid about $8 for each person we brought into the club. The players played for points, which got them into large cash-prize games. Neil and I had a lot of fun, made many friends, and ran poker better than the other four main competitors. We took a salary and little else. We ended up selling the company to our largest competitor.

I spent a couple more years involved in property developments until my daughter was in university and on her own. Scaling down to part-time work, I moved to Brisbane.

With time on my hands and my aunt getting on in years, I had the idea to write her a short sanitized history of my life. Most had been in Europe and very little time spent with her.

Maybe she would be interested. I told her what I was about to do and got busy writing the history.

I received her reply emphatically stating she was, 'not interested, would not read it, and do not send it'.

After she died, I rewrote the story, the explicit version, and sent it to a publisher I had found online and based in Western Australia. Her answer was much the same, 'no woman would ever buy this ego macho crap'.

My days of thinking about being a writer were over until years later, in 2015, I found what I had written. I was now not working except for playing poker, which had earned me about $40,000 in 2014. I reread the story with interest. It was part of my life but there was much more to it than what I had in front of me. Why not write the whole story from the beginning up to when I had enough. Write what actually happened. If I offended anyone, so be it. It had actually happened. There would be no revenge or malice, just the facts. I got into it. Day after day, the story poured out of me. There was no concern for correct structure, spelling that spellcheck couldn't cope with or how to write a book. The focus was to get it down on paper then worry about the other bits later.

My ability to recall events surprised me. I took a trip to the US and spoke to friends I had not seen in many years, to ask questions as to how certain events unfolded. They corrected some of my recollections. I updated the book. By June, I had reached the year 1992 just after I moved to Maui. I thought that was a good place to end the book. It was a point where my life had changed dramatically. Maybe someday I would write another book about what happened in the following years.

I was fortunate to know a talented person who agreed to read the book and edit it for me. Her background and capabilities were perfect for this. She also engaged a friend of hers to recheck her work and then she would go over it again. They both enjoyed doing it. Neither thought it was 'crap' but an exciting story, hard to put down. I was thrilled.

What to do now? I had no idea about the publishing business or how it worked. None! That had never stopped me in the past so I kept going. My thinking had always been, if you don't know how to do something, find someone who does. Pay them well and succeed. If you want to publish a book, get a publisher. I looked online and settled for Australian book publishers located in Brisbane. I wanted to be able to talk face-to-face and understand what was involved.

I met with the woman who ran the company, an author herself. She turned me over to her employee, 'my personal agent', to look after me. I explained about the book. She told me I needed to write a synopsis of the first five chapters. She asked about a cover and I told her I had an idea to use a photo of me. She said they would use it to do the cover for me. They would format the book in e-book and paperback and put it online on Amazon. No editing included, the price would be $1,105 and I would have to sign a contract for a year with them. They would support me with the book during this time and take a percentage of the sales. I thought it was a correct price as I was eager to get my book in print.

For another $400, they would be happy to do a marketing plan for me. I agreed. I was wise enough to know that you needed marketing to sell. They would send the plan to me once the invoice was paid. The book was due to be published in two months. It would take that long to produce the cover, format the book and make any necessary changes. I signed and walked away feeling I was about to be a published author.

The $400 marketing plan arrived as a two-page outline saying that I needed a website. If I wanted them to do it, another $800. I would need to be on Twitter, Facebook, and other social media sites and I should have some business cards printed.

Marketing plan my ass! I made an appointment and went back. Much of what 'my personal agent' had told me was not happening. She said that was their plan. I had to do the work. I told her I had no idea how Twitter worked.

She said, "Learn."

She had seen there were A-listers in my book and wanted them mentioned on the cover. I told her absolutely not. I would not ride on the backs of friends and people I knew to sell my books. This became an argument. Naming known people might sell books. Was I stupid not to use them? I held my ground and left with a bad taste in my mouth.

The book was published in September 2015. I had help from a friend and built a web site: jackkregasbooks. I learned to almost use Twitter. I posted on Facebook. I did understand that without a vast network of followers, this media was not going to have any effect in selling books. It would take time to accumulate followers. None of the promises from the publisher was forthcoming so they were NO help at all. I arranged a meeting with the owner to complain about my agent and her lack of help. I learned that she had been fired for misleading clients.

My reaction was that it didn't surprise me. I explained that her company and I were not a good mix. I wanted out of my twelve-month contract, as promises had not been meet. I felt that now I had more knowledge of how the industry worked, I had been overcharged. The only thing that I was satisfied with was the work done on the cover.

We went around and around until I convinced her that it was in her best interests to let me out of the contract in two weeks, as of October 2015. She could keep the sales until then. If not, her company would appear daily on Facebook and in ads I took out in the local paper informing everyone that they were scam artists, and defrauding their clients. I left the office. Two days later, she emailed me a release.

THEY WERE VANITY PUBLISHERS. BEWARE OF THEM. NEVER USE THEM!

I learned a lesson and thought of an old adage. If you want something done right, do it yourself. With the help of the woman who edited the book and createspace, we learned how to format correctly and had the book on Amazon as self-published before I took the book down from the vanity scammers. Formatting this book with forty photos was more difficult than with a book with no photos. It is not impossible and anyone can learn to do both e-books and paperbacks.

It was now clear to me that writing is the easy part. Selling the book or marketing it is the hard part. I am good face-to-face but online is a new game. Teaching old dogs new tricks is possible! Never think your friends or family will buy or read your books. They may not. If they do, then you're lucky. I asked myself the question, 'who would buy my book?' I am an unknown nobody. I thought if sixty percent of the hundreds of the women I had slept with bought it, and one-half of their boyfriends or ex-husbands in or out of their lives bought it, hey, I would be on my way. They might want to see if they were mentioned and what I had said. I emailed, posted notices, and called friends telling them about the book. The book sold. Reviews came in. Great reviews. People called me. One ex-wife has never spoken to me again.

I never thought of myself as an author and still don't today even after publishing nine books. I am a storyteller. Bullshitting, as I had done all my life to anyone who would listen, but now in print.

Since **IT'S ALL ABOUT ME AND A FEW OTHERS** was *self-published* in November 2015 it has sold steadily, has over fifty, five-star reviews, and sold in twelve countries. An interesting point that made me laugh was that over sixty-five percent of the buyers were women. What do publishers know?

While It's All About Me And A Few Others was being edited and during the time I was learning my lesson with the vanity publisher, I started writing a new book. A novel about euthanasia involving characters everyone can relate too. The more I got into, it the more I liked these characters and their challenges. The book is **CHOICE CRUISE LINES**. I found the man who worked for Australian book publishers to do the cover. The company had moved or changed their name. He no longer had anything to do with them. He did the cover for me for $285. It was published in time for Christmas 2015. This book now has a different cover and is in its third edition. It remains my favorite book.

Many have asked how I write a book and how am I able to do it in six weeks or less. I have an idea, sit down, and write on the computer. I have no outline, no plot ideas, or an ending. There is just the beginning. It develops as I go. If I get stuck, I think about it when I go to bed and usually have an answer by the morning. I don't look to see how others write or think about how someone else might handle the situation. I write what comes into my head.

Here is an example of what I do. When I get up in the morning, I don't have the day planned. I eat something. Maybe a friend calls and says let's meet in the afternoon. Maybe the dog gets sick. Maybe it's a nice day and I decide to go to the beach. On the way home, I stop and eat three tacos and drink two beers. A guy runs into my car in the parking lot. He says it's your fault and gets mad and wants to fight. I kick him in the balls. He goes down. I drive off. Once back at home, I watch TV and go to bed. None of these things were planned. They happened and I reacted.

That is how I write. The character or characters in my books are like me. They do what they have to do in a situation. No planning, just reacting. One event leads them to the next. Of course, imagination and experience helps to add depth to the story. I never think, 'is it good enough?' If it pleases me, that's enough. The editors will fix the spelling and run-on sentences. My job is to get the story on paper.

In 2016, I wrote three books. The second part of my life, **IT'S NOT ONLY ABOUT ME,** covered the period from near where the first book ended, 1992 to 2012. It was very different to the first book in that now I was a single parent living in Australia with responsibilities, something I had tried to avoid all my life.

Because of playing poker, I decided to write about poker. My idea was a story about a man who found some glasses that could see through cards. That was the storyline until it took a turn into a stalker novel and introduced the reluctant hero, Joey Moretti. The more I wrote the more I liked Joey. As soon as **MYSTICAL GLASSES** was completed and published, I wrote **INNOCENT RETRIBUTION,** the second of the Joey Moretti novels.

It was taking me about six to eight weeks to write a novel, depending on how much I traveled or how much I worked. I could write faster than the editors could edit. I designed the cover for Mystical Glasses and my usual man put the design together. The price was now $450. It was costing me far more to produce the books than I was earning from them. It was time for some changes.

I feel a cover should represent the story in the book. Since I know the stories better than anyone, I come up with the ideas for the covers. For some, I have used my own photos but photos are also available online by the thousands. You have only to search to find the one you want to use for your cover. The price for a photo is around $13 or a little more but that allows up to 500,000 uses until you have to pay more.

I then found Fiverr.com, an online company that is a freelance services marketplace. I found a photo for the cover of Innocent Retribution and sent it to a person from Fiverr who made a few requested changes, formatted the cover and sent me 3D photos and banners, all for less than $50. I was saving hundreds on the cover, without sacrificing quality and having exactly what I wanted within five days.

Now I had published five books. The number of my followers on social media was increasing and I had learned how to improve sales online. I also learned that social media, Facebook, Twitter, Instagram, etc, DOES NOT SELL BOOKS. You sell yourself with posts that interest followers. Slipping in a post about your latest book now and then sells a few books. Buying ads from Twitter, Amazon, Google, and the hundreds of 'experts' selling you deals to make your book number one are for the most part a waste of money. I repeat, they are a waste of money, especially when looking at the cost in comparison to the increase, if any, in sales revenue.

Some may disagree with me. If they have found a way to make it work, I want them to tell me. What does work are markets, retirement villages, bookstore signings and anytime you can talk to readers face-to-face and sign your book for them. To sell books you must talk to readers. Social media is a shotgun approach hitting everyone but your market of readers. Find your niche market and work it to death.

A couple of tips on book signings. Unless you are well known or been highly publicized in the area, signing books is not enough to get people into the store. You need to create a reason for them to be there. Advertise that you are giving a lecture to those who are thinking about writing a book. Other topics are how to self-publish or what covers work and why. Give people a reason to come and hear what you have to say. Have your books well presented, and refer to them during your talk. You have a book-interested audience who, with some encouragement, will buy a signed copy of your book.

It is also a good idea to do book signings with one or two other authors. Choose authors who write books that are in a different niche or genre to yours. It gives choice to those who come, as well as a larger audience. Insure the venue where you are doing the signing is prepared to advertise and promote for you. You can do your part but they must do theirs.

How about bookstores in your local area? Will they take your books? I've had my books in six stores in the US and Australia. Most stores will not take Indie authors but that doesn't mean you shouldn't try. Independent bookstores are the best shot. Also, bookstores that only sell Indie authors are springing up in many parts of the world. Find them and get your books on their shelves.

Putting them on the shelf is often the easiest part. Selling them out is the problem. Unless someone in the store pushes your books, they will not move. Soon they take up space where books that sell could be and you will be asked to remove yours. The best way to avoid this is to do book signings at the store or befriend one of the workers. Marketing never sleeps. It is always there and needing your attention.

Now that I had some idea of how the publishing business worked and I had a selection of books to present, I decided to look into finding a major publisher like Random House or Harper Collins Co. I learned there are two main ways to go about this. One is you write a query letter and send it to publishers who are interested in the kind of book you are submitting. According to the professionals who are out there and ready to help you, for a small fee of course, the query letter has to be formatted and perfect to be considered. There are also free sites that guide you in writing this all-important letter.

The second method is to engage a literary agent to approach the publishers for you and present your work. Again, you must convince the agent you have interesting material or be willing to pay the agent to take you on. One I contacted wanted $4,500 to represent me and take fifteen percent of all sales. There was NO guarantee he that he would be successful.

I asked friends I'd made on social media if they had experience in this area. Some found publishers and were happy. Most related they were not happy. Future sales must cover the publisher's expenses and your advance. This means the advance is probably all you'll ever see. Generally, they don't promote and if they do, you may be charged. The main bitch was that the publishers wanted to redo the cover, re-edit the book and/or make changes that the authors were not able to live with. Some who have had publishers told me they got out of their contract so they were free to make all the decisions about their work.

I'm not advising one way or the other, simply passing on general information I have learned. I am sure that many have found publishers and are selling books. I suggest you look very closely before you make any decision. For me, I have decided to continue as an Indie author until an offer too good to refuse comes along.

In 2016, I booked a cruise from LA to Miami through the Panama Canal stopping in numerous places in Mexico and Central America. The canal is 'a must see'. The visits to the small villages and towns in Mexico inspired me to write about them. When I returned home, I wrote the third book in the Joey Moretti series, **CONTESTED RANSOM,** a shootout based mostly in Mexico. Again, I designed the cover and sent it to Fiverr. They also did a video, my first, for the book. By now, I had acquired a following who bought my books and pushed the new release into the top one hundred for a couple of weeks.

While Contested Ransom was being edited, I had an idea to do a book of short stories. There were tales spinning around in my head looking for an exit. Having never considered short stories before, I was eager to try. **TALL TALES** was the result. I put up my idea for the cover on Facebook asking for opinions. A very kind person sent it back with some clever changes and it was the design I used. Making friends on Facebook is important.

Tall Tales included three unrelated stories and a bonus story called MORRIS MORRIS. This story was a give-away on Instafreebie to increase my email list. It worked, with over six hundred new email addresses received. Tall Tales became my second biggest selling book after my autobiography. Fiverr did the video for this book and all the cover posters. I think readers like short stories because they take less time to read in a world where time is in short supply.

DECISIVE SUNSET was my third book in 2017 and my eighth in less than three years. It was also the last in the Joey Moretti series. Joey was now over sixty and had rendered his kind of justice on all the bad guys. He needed a rest, although I was sad to see him retire.

In those three years, I had learned a lot. Unfortunately, all that knowledge won't help sell books in the numbers you hope for. You write not for money, but because you like doing it. Those who contact you or put up a good review, make up for the lack of cash rewards.

I mentioned giving away a short story on Instafreebie for email addresses. This opens up a sensitive subject and one where I have a definite opinion. I send emails to all the addresses I acquired when I gave away that short story, telling them what is happening in my life and announcing the release of a new book. I am not giving anything away. I am not offering a FREE book. Every time, the major response was to unsubscribe. If nothing free is offered, they are not interested.

I gave away two hundred copies of Mystical Glasses and for my efforts found no evidence of selling a book or receiving a review. My research tells me this is, in fact, normal. People who jump on free books are collectors and never read them, and very seldom, if ever, put up a review.

Many authors give away their books with the hope they will be read and a new reader found who will buy a book from them in the future. If you only have one book, the chance of a sale has been given away. It may work if you have many books or a series and the give-away is similar to giving samples of new products to taste and tempt for repeat business. Some have told me that they have had success with this.

My view is that authors and other artists should be paid for their work. A car wash is not free. Your friend, the gardener, charges. Books are an investment in time for the author as well as the costs for publishing them. Giving books away lowers their value in the sense that many think, if it's free, it is inferior. Occasionally I will give books to libraries or as one-on-one promotional material where I can see a return. I do not give away books, not even to family or friends. They should support me by buying and reviewing them.

I have shared my views online and been criticized more than once. With free books everywhere, there is an increase in the mindset of why buy when, if I look, I can get it free. Author's bitch they don't make any money yet continue to give away books. Is giving away one hundred books and gaining one, two or three sales, a success?

I have run promotions where if someone buys the book I am promoting, I will give them another book of mine in e-book form. They have to purchase one to get one free. I am okay with that but I will admit it doesn't work very well. People buy what they want whether it's books or anything else. The ones who search for anything free were never going to pay anyway.

I have spent most of 2018 traveling to research a new book and promote my books when and wherever possible. I print business cards with pictures of the book covers on one side and information about my website and Amazon links on the other. I hand them out anytime anyone shows any interest or asks me what I do. The cards are in full color printed by Vista Print who offer very good prices for cards and other promotional goods.

I spent six months away from writing to give the editors and myself a break. I missed the writing. Normally I start at about 10:00 am and write until 3:00 pm with plenty of timeouts for coffee, ice-cream cones, various other snacks, and sometimes-welcome disruptions. On an average day, I will write 2,500 to 3,000 words without effort. If nothing comes to mind or I don't know where the story is going I stop and start again the next day after having time to think about it. There is no stress or pressure to do anything. Writing is fun. I engage with the characters. They often make me laugh.

The locations I use are real as I have been to most of the places in my books. Equipment, weapons, and cars are researched with the characters using the proper gear for whatever job is at hand. I have fired most of the weapons described in my books. I believe the more true-to-life a situation is described, the more a reader will be involved.

If police or army officers read about an incident in one of my novels, the weapons used are the same as the weapons they would choose. Fiction made to read as fact is far more engaging to me. I think I have this perception because of writing an autobiography as my first book. It was true to life, explicit and real. Knowing actions really happened engages the reader. I continue to write fiction as close to the truth as my imagination allows.

In August 2018, I started a new novel with a new hero, Slick Morrison. Slick was introduced in two of the Joey Moretti novels. He learned from Joey, admiring the way he dealt with people who needed attention. **SLICK JUSTICE** was published in October 2018 to the biggest presale I had ever had, possibly because I had time to plan it with a video and ads. I have mentioned most ads do not work. A company, BooksGoSocial located in Ireland, run by Laurence O'Bryan has been very helpful to me. Laurence always answers my questions and offers advice. I have run ads with him. Some work, some not as well. I still use them because they are fair with the author's interest at heart. If you are an author, I highly recommended being part of this group.

All the time I was writing Slick Justice, I had some new ideas for another book of short stories. I had also experienced a traumatic event I wanted to share with others hoping it might save them some agony in the future. As this story was true, I decided that all the tales should be of a true or advisory nature.

The day Slick headed to the editors, I started on **TALL TALES TWO.** If you are reading this, you already know what has preceded this entry. I decided to include this advice for authors at the last minute simply because so many people ask me the questions I have tried to answer.

I will now try to answer some other questions frequently asked of me.

People at signings and other occasions ask me, 'How do you start? 'Where do you get the ideas?' 'What if no one likes it?'

Let's eliminate the third question first. You cannot please everyone. Please yourself. Write because it is what YOU want to do. Get it on paper. The rest can be taken care of after that.

Start with the idea in your head and write about it as if you're telling the story to a good friend. You will be surprised how easy that will be. Your invisible friend will ask you questions so you answer them and carry on. Before you know it, you have a couple of chapters.

Then there are the more technical questions. 'How many rewrites do you do?' 'What if you don't like the editor's changes?' 'I know nothing of marketing. What do I do?' Then the last question. 'What if no one buys my book?'

The fact is that most Indie authors do not sell one hundred books per month; not one hundred books per year; not one hundred books **EVER!!!** That's right, not one hundred books in their lifetime. If you have published more than one book, of course you may sell more. If you are on Amazon, Draft2Digital, Smash words and many other sites, you **may** sell more. Setting up your website with proper links to these sellers, if you have enough visits, it could improve your sales. The answer is if you are in it to make money, buy a lottery ticket. Your odds are better.

There are any number of internet gurus wanting to teach you marketing and promoters offering to get the word out for you. Be very careful. Learn all you can without spending any money. Take all the freebies (these are 'come-ons') but send no money. I have and it was a waste. Forget about being a bestseller and write another book.

You have to have trust your editor to make the necessary changes while keeping the text in the style you are trying to represent. I admit I am lucky. A man who knew me years ago and read my books told me reading them was just like listening to me telling him stories. That tells me I have editors who are at one with me. Editors can be expensive, up to five cents a word or $10 for a thousand words, if you are lucky. Ask around and find a teacher or a highly trained personal assistant who might be willing to give it a go. Try them with a few chapters and check what they've done. This sample can give you the confidence to continue building the relationship.

The question of rewrites interests me. I have read that some authors spend more time on rewrites than on the book itself. The 2,500 words I write on a Tuesday, I reread before I write anything on Wednesday. I make corrections and never look at it again. I have never read one of my books after it has been edited. On occasion, the editors will ask questions regarding characters, timelines, duplications or sayings that need interpretation. Together we work out what changes to make. My editors patiently make improvements to spelling, punctuation and any twisted grammar. Other than that, I don't try to make it better. I am happy how I told it the first time because I am not trying to be perfect. I'm not perfect so why should my writing be!

Another question that comes up from time to time is, 'what do you think when you get a bad review?'

Everyone wants five-star reviews. Sometimes, you get a one-star review. From what I read online, this shatters some people. I have been fortunate to receive only one bad review. Remember I said that you couldn't please everyone all the time. If the review provides constructive criticism, take it on board to help improve future work. However, because reviewing is an online process, it is open to trolls and other internet nasties. If the review doesn't sound related to your book, forget it and move on. Most of my reviews, which you can see on Amazon US, UK, or Australia have been in the four and five star range.

Reviews are not the only way that you receive criticism. I take it all in. If it is valid, I accept it, if not I forget it. I have been told more than once that my stories end suddenly or it appears that I'm in a hurry to end it. Guilty! I do that. As I have said, I write as if I am telling a story. In describing what happened at dinner I do NOT go into the pattern on the plates. I stick with what is happening.

My style is easy to read. I write to entertain, not to keep someone awake at night trying to figure out what I meant or if there is a hidden meaning. Abrupt endings makes one think about what might have happened or how they would have ended the story. They leave a question. I sometimes do it on purpose or the character says he has had enough. I always do as the characters ask. They are my friends.

Art, photos, books or dishes in a gourmet restaurant appeal to each individual's taste. What one likes, another hates. An artist's job is first to make people know that he or she exists and then hope that some of those like what he or she does. I don't try to be better than someone else. I do try to entertain whoever decides to read one of my books and I hope he or she will read another one and tell their friends. It is a slow process unless you get lucky. I am content if I build up a following for my books one reader at time.

Last words! Please, whenever you read a book by any author, remember to put up a review on Amazon and/or Goodreads. It's the best way to show your appreciation.

www.ingramcontent.com/pod-product-compliance
Lightning Source LLC
Chambersburg PA
CBHW021407210526
45463CB00001B/248